# AIM YOUR
# BRAIN®
## at USMLE Step 1

# AIM YOUR BRAIN®

## at USMLE Step 1

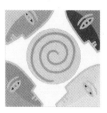

*The Ultimate System for*
*Mastering Multiple-Choice Exams*

**Mary K. Miller, Pharm. D., M.D.**
Foreword by Faith T. Fitzgerald, M.D.

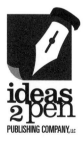

**ideas 2 pen**
PUBLISHING COMPANY, LLC

AIM YOUR BRAIN® at USMLE Step 1
*The Ultimate System for*
*Mastering Multiple-Choice Exams*
Copyright ©2009 by Mary K. Miller, Pharm.D., M.D.

**Ideas2Pen Publishing Company, LLC**
**548 Market Street, Suite 57563**
**San Francisco, CA 94104**
**www.ideas2pen.com**
**info@ideas2pen.com**

Cover and book design by Michael Brechner / Cypress House
Cover illustration: Jose Ortega / Stock Illustration Source/Getty Images

**Note**

Every effort has been made to contact the copyright holders of all photographs and quoted materials. The publisher apologizes for any errors or omissions, and would be grateful for notification of any corrections that should be incorporated into future reprints or editions of this book.

All trademarks are trademarks of their respective owners. Rather than put a trademark symbol after every occurrence of a trademarked name, we use names in an editorial fashion only, and to the benefit of the trademark owner, with no intention of infringement of the trademark. Specific trademarks owned by Dr. Miller are AIM YOUR BRAIN® and F.A.C.T.O.I.D.®. The AIM YOUR BRAIN® Study System is patent pending.

Publisher's Cataloging-in-Publication Data

Miller, Mary K., 1951-
   AIM YOUR BRAIN® at USMLE Step 1 : the ultimate system for mastering multiple choice exams / by Mary K. Miller, Pharm.D., M.D. -- 1st ed.
-- Sacramento, CA : Ideas2Pen Publishing, LLC, 2009.
(AIM YOUR BRAIN®)
   ISBN: 978-0-9821343-4-4
Includes index.
   1. Medicine--Examinations--United States--Study guides.
2. Physicians--Licenses--United States--Examinations--Study
guides. 3. Study skills--United States. 4. Examinations--Study
guides. I. Title. II. United States medical licensing examination.
III. AIM YOUR BRAIN®.
   R834.5 .M55 2009                            2008944245
   610.76--dc22 0906
First edition

Printed in the USA
2 4 6 8 9 7 5 3 1

# Disclaimer

The information contained in this study system and related materials including but not limited to any marketing materials, promotional materials and any handouts or other materials as well as any information provided in any seminars, lectures or other presentations related to such information ("Information" herein, individually, jointly, and collectively) is based on information from sources believed to be accurate and reliable and every reasonable effort has been made to make the Information as complete and accurate as possible but such completeness and accuracy cannot be guaranteed and is not guaranteed. The reader and user of the Information should use the Information as a study guide only and only as part of the reader's and user's other study materials and not rely solely on the Information. The author, the publisher, and any other party are not engaged in the rendering of medical, psychological, pharmacological, or other advice as a result of writing or publishing or otherwise making the Information available.

The Information is provided on an "as is" basis without any warranties, express or implied, of any kind, whether warranties as to use, merchantability, fitness for a particular purpose, or any other warranties. Without limiting the generality of the foregoing, the author and the publisher do not warrant or represent that any of the Information shall be successful in helping the reader or user pass any examination, licensing test, or otherwise, or achieve any particular score on any of the same. The author and the publisher shall not be liable to the reader and user or any other party for any direct or indirect compensatory, special, incidental, or consequential damages or costs of any character including but not limited to damages or costs for the acts of any other party, and the author and the publisher shall not be liable for any damages or costs in excess of the price the reader and user paid for the study system and related materials even if the author and the publisher shall have been informed of the possibility of such damages or costs, or for any claim by any other party. The within exclusions and limitations of warranties may be limited by the laws of certain states or other jurisdictions, and so some of the foregoing exclusions and limitations may not apply to the reader and user, and the reader and user may have other rights that may vary from state to state.

If the reader and user do not agree with any of the terms of the foregoing, the reader and user should *not* read this study system or related materials and should immediately return this study system and related materials to the publisher at the address indicated in this study system with the receipt for such purchase and the reader's and user's money will be refunded. If the reader and user do not return this study system and related materials, the reader and user will be deemed to have accepted the provisions of this disclaimer.

*This book is dedicated to the memory of*
*Richard H. Oi, M.D. (1930–2007)*
*Professor Emeritus,*
*Obstetrics & Gynecology and Pathology*
*University of California Davis School of Medicine*

---

*A teacher affects eternity;*
*he can never tell where*
*his influence stops.*

— Henry Adams
*(US author and historian, 1838–1918)*

# Contents

# Foreword

*Personally, I have always been opposed to that base and most pernicious system of educating...with a view to examinations...*

> — William Osler M.D., a 19th-century founder
> of modern American Medical Education

There is a great difference between medical school education (in which students, under expert guidance, craft themselves into knowledgeable, skilled, compassionate, curious, and dedicated scientifically and humanistically capable physicians and investigators) and our standardized evaluations of those students (examinations, generally... and endlessly). But the practical and inescapable point is that passing examinations, as Dr. Miller so clearly explains, is a skill that, while not a true measure of excellence as a doctor, is perpetually required if one wants to be a doctor.

There are many "exam books" a student can buy or borrow that promise improvement in scores on upcoming exams, but few *systems* of approach to multiple choice exams that are life-long brain-training in and of themselves: Dr. Miller has come up with one, and one that both works and endures in usefulness for an entire lifetime in Medicine. Rather as the scientific method is superior to storing up the "scientific facts" of the moment, and the diagnostic thought process better than immediate labeling of patient problems by the most obvious first impression, so too is this "AIM YOUR BRAIN" study system vastly superior to the usual cramming.

Most attractively, it assumes what caring teachers know to be true: Medical students are bright, responsible, gifted men and women who learn in many different ways. Our mutual task, students and their teachers, is to find the way that fits the student best.

Faith T. Fitzgerald, M.D.
Professor, Internal Medicine
Associate Dean of Humanities and Bioethics
UC Davis School of Medicine

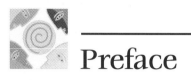

# Preface

*Dear Dr. Miller:*

*I am writing you because I need some help. One of our students has failed her USMLE examination and her first shelf examination. I remembered the good work you've done helping students in similar situations. This student is struggling with her standardized test taking. I know you are very busy, but can you help her get through these hurdles? I would appreciate your considering whether you can fit her into your hectic schedule.*

Signed, Assistant Dean, Office of Medical Education*
(*Paraphrased to protect the innocent.)

Julia and I were off and running. All I had to do was set up an official clinical faculty advisor relationship, arrange a strategy meeting, create a study schedule, identify any learning disabilities, overcome any learning disabilities, help Julia (not her real name) repeat and pass her USMLE Step 1 and NBME "shelf" exams, and get her back in sync to resume her regularly scheduled clerkship rotations. Of course all Julia had to do was... all of the above, and allow me to completely change her study and test-taking methods. The other good news was that we had only a little over three months to pull the whole thing off.

Were we able to do it? Were we successful? Of course we were. Working as a team, Julia and I were able to develop rapport and trust quickly. Because of her openness to change, I was able to implement a system that led to her passing her USMLE Step 1 and clerkship "shelf" exam retakes; and to the passing of *all* subsequent clerkship exams—on the *first try*.

Since working with Julia, and others before her, I've continued to help more and more students. What I'm finding is that when it comes to putting my study system into practice, I keep repeating the same things to each new student. Granted, I'm trying to focus my techniques to each one's particular situation, and of course get to know them, but the basic approach is the same for most students.

One afternoon, between rushing off to clinic to see patients and sitting in my office thinking about what else I needed to do to help one of my students, the light bulb went on in my mind and I said, "Okay, that does it. I'm writing this book!"

Julia is one person representing thousands of students who are accomplished, bright, and talented, but have difficulty passing timed multiple-choice tests. I guess I've become, by default, the "go-to" faculty person who now specializes in helping individuals learn the specific skill set that enables them to pass these exams so that they can become doctors. But, in my heart, I don't feel like this is something I'm obligated to do; I *want* to help my students. My problem is that there's just one of me, and I need to reach more students.

Call me old-fashioned, but I believe in commitment. It seems that we work so hard to pick students to come to our medical schools all over the country, and then if they have problems—not because they're not intelligent or hardworking, but because of this issue with taking timed multiple-choice exams—we're so quick to penalize them. We're almost too ready to jettison them off to the ice floe, to kick them out. This has always rubbed me the wrong way. I don't understand it. If you have a student who isn't working or just doesn't have it, well, that's a different story. But I'm seeing the same kind of students over and over again: They're bright, they're hardworking, they care, and they have the potential to be fabulous physicians. They hit this bump in the road that is absolutely devastating to them, and embarrassing, and they don't know what to do. They experience self-doubt, and they feel immense shame; they don't want anyone to know they have failed. This isn't just a problem at my school; it's a problem at many if not most schools.

I decided I had to do something, so I began to create a system to help my students succeed. Our institutions of medical education accomplish so much in so little time, but we're not necessarily building in other skill sets that our students need. Since the whole game of medical licensure has to do primarily with taking timed multiple-choice exams, I don't think we're focused enough on helping medical students who have trouble getting through them.

So here we are. Now that this book is done, the big question is: what's in it for you? What are you going to learn from this book?

You're going to learn:

- How to prepare for, pass, or retake your USMLE Step 1 exam, depending on your specific situation;

- That there are historical reasons for these exams, and like it or not, they're not going away.

- Most of you hate multiple-choice exams, but you've got to get over that and let me help you figure out a way to get through the maze.

- The key to helping you prepare for and pass your Step 1 Exam is learning how to use the AIM YOUR BRAIN Study System.

- The key to really passing these exams is to also identify potential obstacles—major test anxiety, learning disabilities, etc.—early, rather than later, and doing something about them.

I know you're busy. I know you're thinking, *I don't even have time to handle my current workload, much less read this book, study it, and do the exercises. Why do I even have to do this?* Well, for some of you, the answer is scary, but it's simple. If you don't do something now, you may get kicked out of medical school. For the rest of you, the time has come to try a different approach. If you don't change the way you prepare for your "board" exams, then you're going to find yourself in the same predicament that led you to buy this book in the first place. It's really a vicious cycle: Take the test, fail the test, take the test, fail the test. Get called into your school's version of the "Committee on Student Performance." Sink into some form of deep despair. Fear starts to drive your decisions. "What if I fail again? Whom should I tell? What should I do now? Will I graduate? Will any residency program even interview me, let alone rank me?"

Oh, yeah, one more thing: What about the loans? Most students these days, don't go into medicine because of the money, because there's a lot more things you can do (in a lot less time) to make a lot more money. You go into medicine because you want to help people and you love the sciences. The problem is that as you go through medical school, you incur enormous debt. So part of this fear thing has to do with, "If I'm being told I might be kicked out of medical school because of my test scores, exactly what am I supposed to do with the $80,000 or $150,000 or (insert your own number) debt? And by the way, I'm in between careers right now, and I have no way to pay it off."

What a double whammy—you go into a profession knowing that you have other career options, in some cases even better-paying options, and then you run into this type of potentially ego-shattering obstacle. The sense of impending doom is very scary when you start to have problems taking these exams, so there's an urgent need to try to help you stay in medical school.

Someday, there may be a way to change medical-school curricula so as to insure that all students, regardless of their learning style, are ready for these exams. But the intent of this book isn't to change the system; my intent is to help you with the current system, because that's all we have to work with. This book is about giving you what you need to know right now, so that you can pass your test. It should save you a heck of a lot of money, a heck of a lot of time, and a whole lot of hassle.

The style of the book is intentional. It's designed to deliver information in a way that makes it easily digestible and useable. I don't want you to have to carry around another huge, twenty-pound textbook. This book is deliberately small in size so that you really can toss it in your backpack or purse (if you have one). The idea is that I want you to take it with you everywhere you go, so if you have ten minutes here, and ten minutes there, you can dip in and derive value in your downtime. Also, this book is designed to be sensitive to different learning styles; it isn't just left-brain linear—do this—but more user-friendly.

This book will be inspiring as well as instructional. While you're learning how to take these tests by using the AIM

YOUR BRAIN Study System, you'll meet a couple of my students—people just like you—one who faced challenges and successfully overcame the obstacles, and another without academic difficulties who just wanted to find a better way to study for USMLE Step 1.

*Mary K. Miller, Pharm.D., M.D.*

# Acknowledgments

First of all, I would like to thank all of the students who gave me the opportunity to coach and teach them. You inspired me to forge ahead and write this book. I would like to thank Sam Horn for being such a wonderful mentor and teacher and the members of our original Maui Writer's Retreat group: Vera Gilford, Marcie Herring, Hamilton McCubbin, Pat Nordberg, Carol O'Dwyer, Georglyn Rosenfeld, Rick Sheff, Zanna Smith, Victoria Stein, Wendy Trocchio, Cathy Wong, and Kathy Wood. I am eternally grateful to Lloyd Smith, M.D., Ph.D. and Pamela Bigelow for their support and belief in my "coaching" mission. Special thanks to my colleagues at the UC Davis School of Medicine, Dean's Office: Ann Bonham, Ph.D. (Executive Associate Dean, Academic Affairs), Faith Fitzgerald, M.D. (Associate Dean, Ethics and Humanities); Vijaya Kumari, MBBS, Ph.D. (former Associate Dean [interim], Curriculum); and Gail Peoples, M.P.A. (Office of Medical Student Affairs-Academic Support). Also, I would like to acknowledge the incredible work being done every day by: Emil Rodolfa, Ph.D. (Director of the UCD Counseling and Psychological Services-CAPS Program) and his team, Karin Nilsson, Ph.D. and Karen Paez, Ph.D.; Christine O'Dell (UCD Student Disability Center) and Jennifer Grimes, Ph.D., LED (Private Practice-Licensed Educational Psychologist).

As for the editing, typesetting, book-design guidance and production, I would like to thank Cynthia Frank, Joe Shaw,

Michael Brechner, Stephanie Rosencrans, John Fremont, and Sharon Groth of Cypress House. I would like to offer special thanks to my friends Shagufta Yasmeen, M.D., Marion Jones, R.N., N.P., and Cathy Zampa, R.N. for their unwavering support. Finally, loving thanks to Judith Franks, who believed in this book project from beginning to end and also believed in the writer.

# CHAPTER 1

## USMLE's First Step

*A journey of a thousand miles begins with a single step.*

— Lao Tzu (604 BC–531 BC)

## What Is USMLE Step 1?

To make sure everyone is on the same page, let's begin by reviewing a few things. As you probably know by now, USMLE is an acronym that stands for the United States Medical Licensing Examination. USMLE Step 1 is the first part of a three-part series of written exams; it focuses on the things you learned during your first two years of medical school, i.e., basic sciences. In addition to Step 1, there are two more exams, Step 2 and Step 3, which focus on the clinical sciences. There is also a clinical-skills portion known as Step 2 CS (clinical skills). You must pass each of the written exams and the clinical-skills portion for licensure in the United States. Of course, there may be additional requirements for different states, and these can vary from jurisdiction to jurisdiction. You'll need to check this out prior to applying for licensure in your state.

You may be wondering how this licensing thing came to be. The short answer is that you can thank Dr. William Rodman for moving to Philadelphia from Kentucky in the late 1800s.[1] Believe it or not, there's a real story to this whole licensure deal, and it's included in appendix 1 at the back of this book.

## NBME and USMLE

NBME stands for the National Board of Medical Examiners, which was founded in 1915.[1] So as not to hold you up as you peruse the first few chapters of this book, the beginning of the NBME also had something to do with Dr. Rodman. Of course the details can be found in appendix 1.

The USMLE Step series has been morphed from the original weeklong endurance exam, via essays and bedside oral practical exams, to the computerized versions we have today.[1] Nowadays, the NBME and USMLE work together to get medical students through the medical licensure maze. If you want to know more details, go to—you know—appendix 1.

## Registration Entities? NBME and ECFMG

On the USMLE.org website there's a chart that shows two pathways to registration for Step 1. One is to sign up on the NBME website, and the other is via the ECFMG website (Educational Commission for Foreign Medical Graduates). Essentially, if you're a student or graduate of a medical school in the United States or Canada that is accredited by the LCME or AOA (here we go again, more acronyms: Liaison Committee on Medical Education or the American Osteopathic Association) then you register via www.Nbme.org. If you're a student or graduate of a medical school outside the US and Canada, then you must register using www.Ecfmg.org.

The ECFMG has a very interesting history of its own. It was started in 1956 to help address the shortage of physicians in the United States. After World War II, there was increased demand for healthcare services and not enough US-trained physicians to fill the need. Physicians from other countries came to the US to work. Since there was no formal evaluation and certifying process available for international medical school graduates, one was created.

A bunch of organizations with lots of acronyms—the Association of American Medical Colleges (AAMC), the American Hospital Association (AHA), the Federation of State Medical Boards (FSMB), and the American Medical Association (AMA)—formed the Cooperating Committee on Graduates of Foreign Medical Schools (CCGFMS) in 1954.[2] The CCGFMS ultimately became the ECFMG after a few more variations on the theme (for the precise organizational development please visit the ECFMG website).

So if you're an international medical graduate (IMG), I highly recommend you spend some time at www.Ecfmg.org. The organization just celebrated its "50th Golden Anniversary" and has lots of experience in getting IMGs through the US licensure process.[3]

## Fig. 1.1          Chart Your Course

| | |
|---|---|
| **1. Who is eligible to take Step 1?** | a. Med students enrolled in an accredited US or Canadian MD med school (LCME accredited)<br><br>b. Graduates from an accredited US or Canadian MD med school (LCME accredited)<br><br>c. Med students enrolled in an accredited US DO med school (AOA accredited)<br><br>d. Graduates from an accredited US DO med school (AOA accredited)<br><br>e. Med students enrolled in med school outside of the USA and Canada and eligible for exam by ECFMG<br><br>f. Graduates of med school outside the USA and Canada and eligible for exam by ECFMG |
| **2. When can I take Step 1?** | a. After completing the first two years of an accredited medical school program |
| **3. How do I apply?** | a. US and Canadian med students and graduates of accredited MD and DO schools can apply via the NBME website (www.nbme.org)<br><br>b. Med students and graduates of med schools NOT in the US or Canada can apply via the ECFMG website (www.ecfmg.org)<br><br>c. Check with your school for their suggested time to take Step 1<br><br>d. Pick three-month window of time when you would like to take exam<br><br>e. Once your exam application is approved, you will get your Scheduling Permit good for your 3-month eligibility period<br><br>f. Sign up for an exam appointment at a Prometric Test Center (www.prometric.com) |
| **4. How much does it cost?** | a. US or Canadian med student or graduate is currently ~$495 USD (Can be other fees depending on your situation)<br><br>b. According to ECFMG website: ~$695 USD + other fees |
| **5. Where do I take the exam?** | a. Go to the Prometric website (www.prometric.com) and follow the links to find a center near you |
| **6. Additional questions?** | a. Go to the appropriate website (content is subject to change)    www.nbme.org<br>www.ecfmg.org<br>www.usmle.org<br>www.prometric.com |

Just in case you're not a chart-minded person, I'm putting the chart information in outline form with a little more white space.

1. **Who is eligible to take Step 1?**

   a. Med students enrolled in an accredited US or Canadian MD med school (LCME accredited)

   b. Graduates from an accredited US or Canadian MD med school (LCME accredited)

   c. Med students enrolled in an accredited US DO med school (AOA accredited)

   d. Graduates from an accredited US DO med school (AOA accredited)

   e. Med students enrolled in school outside the US and Canada who are eligible for exam by ECFMG

   f. Graduates of med school outside the US and Canada who are eligible for exam by ECFMG

2. **When can I take Step 1?**

   a. After completing the first two years of an accredited medical school program

3. **How do I apply?**

   a. US and Canadian med students and graduates of accredited MD and DO schools can apply via the NBME website: www.Nbme.org

   b. Med students and graduates of med schools *not* in the US or Canada can apply via the ECFMG website: www.Ecfmg.org

   c. Check with your school for their suggested time to take Step 1

d. Pick the three-month window of time when you would like to take the exam

e. Once your exam application is approved, you'll get your scheduling permit good for your three-month eligibility period

f. Sign up for an exam appointment at a Prometric Test Center: www.prometric.com

## 4. How much does it cost?

a. For US or Canadian med students or graduates the price is currently $495 US (there can be other fees depending on your situation)

b. According to the ECFMG website, it's $695 US + other fees

## 5. Where do I take the exam?

a. Go to the Prometric website (www.prometric.com) and follow the links to find a center near you

## 6. Additional questions?

a. Go to the appropriate website (content is subject to change)

   i. www.Nbme.org

   ii. www.Ecfmg.org

   iii. www.Usmle.org

   iv. www.prometric.com

## Step 1 Preparation and Question Types

I'm sure you're wondering what's on the Step 1 exam. The quick answer is, everything you learned in your first two years of medical school. Just kidding—but sometimes preparing for it feels overwhelming. No one outside of the USMLE and NBME really knows what's on the exam, and that's the way it should be. The USMLE folks do publish an extensive content outline for your review on www.Usmle.org. I list just the highlights below:

1. **General Principles**

    a. Anatomy

    b. Behavioral Stuff

    c. Biochem

    d. Micro

    e. Path

    f. P'Col

    g. Physio

    h. And More

2. **Systems**

    a. Hematopoietic and Lymphoreticular

    b. Nervous and Special Senses

    c. Skin and Connective Tissue

    d. Musculoskeletal

    e. Respiratory

    f. Cardiovascular

    g. Gastrointestinal

    h. Renal/Urinary

    i. Reproductive

    j. Endocrine

**3. Process**

    a. 30–50% Normal Structure and Function

    b. 30–50% Abnormal Processes

    c. 15–25% Principals of Therapeutics

    d. 10–20% Psycho-social, Cultural, Occupational, and Environmental Considerations

Step 1 is designed to test what you learned during your first two years in med school, emphasizing the basic sciences, of course. Remember: As you go through the preparation process, the content and testing approach are subject to change. A good example of this is associating some multiple-choice questions with media clips. Don't panic, you'll have an opportunity to practice using media clips before exam day.

In 1999, the USMLE completed their transition from the old fashion PPT (pen-and-paper test) to the CBT (computer-based-test) in use today. So why the change? It's a lot easier for the test givers—and you as a test taker don't have to wait as long to take it. Step 1 used to be given only a couple times a year.

The computerized format also allows enhanced test security, ease of grading, better access to testing centers, more interesting question types (i.e., clearer images), and faster turnaround in score reporting.

You may be wondering, then, just how you're supposed to prepare for Step 1. Many students just pull together a few review books and class notes, get access to an online question bank, and wait until the last minute. If that's your approach, and if it works for you, then keep it up.

What I've noticed while teaching medical students over the years is that not all of them do well or feel comfortable using this method. I hear it over and over again: "I really studied hard for Step 1 but didn't do as well as I thought I would," or "I just don't do well on multiple-choice exams, and now that I'm in medical school, I don't know what to do. I know I'll be a better doctor than what my scores show."

I don't have all the answers, but I can tell that if you decide to try a different approach to your Step 1 preparation, you *must* separate the clinician from the test taker. You must look at Step 1 for what it is—a timed multiple-choice exam (in spite of the spiffing up).

Becoming a great physician is a process that involves more than this exam: You will acquire knowledge and skills in the classroom and laboratory; at the bedside and in the clinic; in the operating room and in the emergency department, and on labor and delivery. You'll also gain knowledge and skills during your preparation and review for Step 1. You now need to focus on the exam and its content using the tools presented in this book. The next step is yours.

## CHAPTER 2

# "I Hate Multiple-choice Exams"

*Examinations are formidable even to the best prepared, for the greatest fool may ask more than the wisest man can answer.*

— Charles Caleb Colton (1780–1832)

## Have I Told You Today How Much I Hate Multiple-choice Exams?

My apologies to the NBME, USMLE, and all the other alphabet salads. The Colton quote is not meant to be disrespectful to anyone who writes tests or asks hard questions in the classroom or on rounds. The point is that you can never know the answers to all the questions, no matter how smart or well prepared you are. But what you can do is accept this fact and move on. You goal is to do the very best you can on Step 1, and to learn techniques that will help you get through your multiple-choice-question challenges.

As for the name of this chapter, there's a story. Almost every time I met with Julia, we would say our hellos, and then, at the beginning of our session, she would say, "Dr. Miller, have I told you how much I hate multiple-choice questions today?" We would both laugh ... and that became our running joke.

For me the title of this chapter sums up the way many people feel about multiple-choice questions, and exams in general: they either love them or hate them. So we're going to take a little time to actually examine multiple-choice questions and exams and see if we can get you to a place (if you're one of those who hate them) that's a little more tolerable.

## Why Are Multiple-choice Tests Hard For Some People?

Here, according to my students, are the main reasons they dislike multiple-choice tests (code for "find them harder"):

1. They run out of time.

2. They thought they knew the material.

3. They didn't understand the question(s).

4. The correct answer wasn't there.

5 They studied the wrong things.

6. They only got partway through their online question bank.

7. They were distracted.

8. They felt anxiety.

9. They were fatigued.

According to the book *Mastering Multiple Choice* by Stephen Merritt,[4] the reasons people don't do well on multiple-choice tests are (my comments are in parentheses):

1. Overconfidence (obvious)

2. Trickery (as in, question writers think multiple-

choice questions (MCQs) are easy so they try to trick you)

3. Time pressures (again, obvious)

4. Broader range of topics can be covered quickly in MCQ exams

5. Specific data is present (like the right answer), so a greater level of detail may be asked

6. Can't bluff your answers

7. MCQs can be difficult for the question writer to write

8. Content is shuffled (biochemistry is mixed in with pharmacology and pathology, etc.; no separate blocks for each)

So whether you find multiple-choice tests difficult or easy, you need to have a strategy to study for them. You'll learn more about the AIM YOUR BRAIN Study System in chapter 4. For now, just remember that there are methods in this book to help you get through all of this.

## What Is a Multiple-choice Test?

**mul • ti • ple - choice**[5] – adjective

1. consisting of several possible answers from which the correct one must be selected: a multiple-choice question.

2. made up of multiple-choice questions: a multiple-choice exam.

No surprises here. A multiple-choice test is nothing more than an exam made up of multiple-choice questions. Now don't go crazy on me here, I know you knew that—I'm just trying to lay a little foundation, okay?

## Anatomy of A Multiple-choice Question

A multiple-choice question or item (since not all test items are in the form of a question) consists of three parts:

1. the stem, which asks the question, makes a statement, poses a problem involving images, charts, or graphs, or presents a case history, etc.;

2. the correct answer;

3. and four (or more) alternative responses or completions that are incorrect, called distracters.[6, 7]

### Example 1

A twenty-two-year-old woman has just been diagnosed with HIV. She has heard about a new class of medications called integrase inhibitors. Which of the following drugs is an integrase inhibitor? [This is the stem.]

   (A) Lamivudine      [DISTRACTER]

   (B) Raltegravir      [CORRECT ANSWER]

   (C) Ribavirin       [DISTRACTER]

   (D) Rifampin       [DISTRACTER]

   (E) Ritonovir       [DISTRACTER]

## Current USMLE Step 1 Question Types

Only single or individual questions with *one best answer* are included on Step 1. According to the Step 1 Test Question Format found on the USMLE website,

> These items consist of a statement or question followed by three to eleven response options arranged in alphabetical or logical order. A portion of the questions involves interpretation of graphic or pictorial materials. The response options for all questions are lettered (e.g., A, B, C, D, E). Examinees are required to select the best answer to the question. Other options may be partially correct, but there is only *one best answer*.[8]

### Example 2

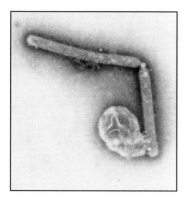

**Fig. 2.1: Influenza A *virions*.[9]**

During August to October 2004, sporadic human cases of bird flu were reported in Vietnam and Thailand. The above transmission electron micrograph (TEM) shows two of the avian influenza *A virions*. What is the influenza A virus subtype of greatest concern for avian flu?

(A) H1N1          [DISTRACTER]

(B) H1N2          [DISTRACTER]

(C) H3N2          [DISTRACTER]

(D) H4N1          [DISTRACTER]

(E) H5N1          [CORRECT ANSWER]

## Example 3

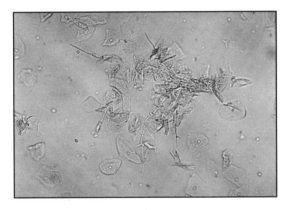

Fig. 2.2: Vaginal
wet mount.[10]

The above wet mount shows what type of infection?

(A) Bacterial vaginosis      [DISTRACTER]

(B) Candida albicans         [CORRECT ANSWER]

(C) *Chlamydia arachomatis*  [DISTRACTER]

(D) *E. coli*                [DISTRACTER]

(E) *Trichomonas vaginalis*  [DISTRACTER]

## Why Does USMLE Step 1 Use Multiple-choice Questions?

As you'll recall from chapter 1, the NBME was founded in 1915. The next year, during October 16–21, 1916, the first examination of the National Board was given. This exam consisted of written, oral, laboratory, and clinical tests.[11]

In 1922, after seeing how things were done in Europe, the NBME divided the old weeklong exam into three parts. Part I was a three-day written essay examination in the basic sciences. Part II was a two-day written essay examination in what is today referred to as the clinical sciences. Part III was a one-day practical oral examination, conducted at the bedside and in the laboratory, on clinical and laboratory problems.[1]

In 1954, the NBME Part I and Part II exams were converted from essays to multiple-choice-question format. Prior to this change, a three-year study was undertaken in which examinations were given that included both essay-type and multiple-choice-formatted questions. The study results showed the "scores derived from the multiple-choice portion of the tests corresponded much more closely with the long-term evaluation of students by their instructors than did the essay test grades."[1]

In Hubbard and Clemans's 1961 book, *Multiple-Choice Examinations In Medicine,* we get a little insight into the thinking at the time after the decision was made to dump the essay questions:

> Confronted with the problems and uncertainties of measuring knowledge, the medical profession—its medical educators and examining boards—is turning more and more to the science of educational measurement and to those skilled in testing techniques.[7]

The examiners new to writing multiple-choice questions wanted to ensure "a greater degree of reliability, comparability, and validity."[7]

By 1971, in another book penned by Dr. Hubbard, the NBME seemed more confident in using multiple-choice exams in assessing physician knowledge and clinical competence.

The measurements of individuals, who are the product of the educational system, may be analyzed and studied collectively for classes of students and groups of physicians at varying points of development, thereby yielding objective assessments of the effectiveness of the educational system. Evaluation of the product thus provides evaluation of the process.[6]

I guess we're all products of the process. I never thought to put it that way... exactly.

In today's technology-based world, it's easy to see how the use of the multiple-choice-question format has made the transformation to computer-based testing (CBT) a reality. Remember: CBT started in 1999 (not that long ago). Some of benefits of CBT are enhanced test security, ease of grading, better access to testing centers, more interesting question types (i.e., clearer images), and faster turnaround in score reporting. So, regarding why USMLE Step 1 uses multiple-choice questions, the simple answer is, to keep up with the times.

## 10 Things You Can Do to Improve Your MCQ Test-taking Skills Regardless of Content

1. **PRACTICE** your computer-based testing skills before you take the test. This will help to reduce anxiety.

2. **READ** the question carefully (no skimming).

3. **ANSWER** first... come up with your own answer and then see if it's in the choices listed. If so, it's probably correct.

4. **LOOK** at each of the responses and read them carefully.

5. **BEWARE** of answers that are true but don't have anything to do with the question topic.

6. **ELIMINATE** the distracters you know are wrong; if you get it down to two choices, you have a 50/50 chance of getting it right.

7. **START** with the questions you can answer easily.

8. **WATCH** your time per block and time per question, and leave a little time at the end of the block to review your answers.

9. **CHANGE** your answer only if you have a really good reason to do so.

10. **GUESS**, if you haven't got a clue and time is running out.

## CHAPTER 3

# Feats of Learning

*Personally I'm always ready to learn, although I do not always like being taught.*

— Sir Winston Churchill (1874–1965)

## Introduction

L earning is an active process. The word "learn" means "to acquire knowledge of or skill in by study, instruction, or experience."[12] The word "feat" is defined as "an act of skill, endurance, imagination, or strength; an achievement."[13] Feats of learning means acquiring knowledge by studying skillfully. The intent of this book is to help you study skillfully and efficiently.

To get to this point in your education, you have learned how to read, write, apply abstract reasoning, solve complex equations, etc. If you're lucky you also gained skills in music, the arts, and sports. You zeroed in on your passion to help others and worked incredibly hard to get into medical school. Along the way you adapted to different teaching styles and subject matter. You've had to make good grades and be successful in class and on paper.

Depending on how your brain is wired, you either found a way to be successful in all forms of testing, i.e., multiple-choice, short answer, oral exams, lab practicals, term papers, scholarly projects, etc., or you made it through not knowing exactly how you did it.

I believe that learning preferences come into play. Depending on whom you read, the preferences are organized as follows:[14, 15]

**1. Somatic or kinesthetic**

**2. Auditory**

**3. Visual**

**4. Intellectual**

If you've read anything on accelerated learning, that's the heart of Dave Meier's SAVI system in his book *The Accelerated Learning Handbook*. SAVI is the first letter of each of the learning preferences listed above.

Some educators think learning preferences, or styles, don't really exist. I don't take such a hard line. In the coaching I've done with medical students, using the idea of learning preferences has provided a framework and a starting point to aid in revamping and reorganizing failed approaches to Step 1 study.

As you've probably gathered by now, I like to change things around so they're easier to remember and more applicable to my teaching style. Think of the following as "learning tags." Simply put, how do you learn best? Do you learn best by:

**Sight:** The power or faculty of seeing; perception of objects by use of the eyes; vision.[16]

**Sound:** The sensation produced by stimulation of the organs of hearing by vibrations transmitted through the air or other medium.[17]

**Motion:** The action or process of moving or of changing place or position; movement.[18]

**Muse:** To think or meditate in silence, as on some subject.[19]

Or do you learn by a combination of some or all of the above? In the next sections I'll elaborate on each learning preference and help you identify how you learn best. Finally, I'll encourage you to try a study-style makeover and see if you might be able to try a slightly different approach to studying for Step 1.

## Learning Tags: Sight, Sound, Motion, and Muse

According to Wikipedia, the free encyclopedia, "A tag is a (relevant) keyword or term associated with or assigned to a piece of information (e.g., a picture, article, or video clip), thus describing the item and enabling keyword-based classification of information."

I want you to think about how you would "tag" yourself. I realize that tagging yourself may seem weird, but give it a try anyway. Examples of each tag with a little more description include:

- **Sight learning** emphasizes seeing, observing, and mind mapping (think looking at a video, through a microscope, or at a chart).

- **Sound learning** emphasizes hearing, listening, and talking (think lectures, audio programs, etc.).

- **Motion learning** emphasizes moving and hands-on experiences (think tying knots, handling surgical instruments, etc.).

- **Muse learning** emphasizes thinking, problem solving, and planning (think scientific method, or pondering a specific question, etc.).

The tags for sight, sound, motion, and muse should elicit some kind of response in you such as "Oh, I'm a lecture person. If I hear it once, I can remember it, no problem. I respond to sound." Another example might be "I love to think about things, work a problem in my mind, contemplate. I guess I would tag myself as 'muse.'"

The point of all of this is to help you identify how you've been learning up to this point. It doesn't matter whether you lean toward one tag or a combination of all four. It's something you need to "muse" about. Because once you're consciously aware of how you learn, you have an opportunity to experiment with the other ways. Studying for multiple-choice exams can be boring. In later chapters you'll see how knowing your "tag" and being open to trying other learning techniques can help you in your Step 1 preparation.

## Step By Step, "Putting It Together"

In Stephen Sondheim's musical *Sunday In The Park With George,* the characters sing the song *Putting It Together* as they discuss the difficulties of putting an artistic enterprise together and the steps it takes to do it. This book is intended to help you "put it together" and pass your Step 1 enterprise—I mean exam.

The next chapters are designed to help you to maximize your learning preference(s) or tags. Many of my students have rediscovered former approaches to learning that they unknowingly discarded in the past. They assumed they were "putting it together" because the learning style(s) they were using prior to medical school worked fine when they were in college. They now realize that medical school isn't "undergrad," and that it may take a different strategy to succeed.

So, now that you know something about your learning preferences, here is the good news and the bad news as they apply to studying for Step 1 and the AIM YOUR BRAIN Study System The good news is, if you're inclined toward sight, sound, or motion, there are specific things you can do that will help you get through your online question banks and F.A.C.T.O.I.D. book(s) review. F.A.C.T.O.I.D. is an acronym for "Frequently Asked Concepts To Own In Depth," and a F.A.C.T.O.I.D. book is the spiral-bound notebook you create for those concepts that are giving you trouble.

If you're more of a "muser," you'll have to expand your horizons and add sight, sound, or both skills to your repertoire, and reduce your musing time while studying for Step 1. If you muse your way through your review, you'll probably run out of time without finishing the AIM YOUR BRAIN Study System. If you must muse, then set a specific amount of time per day—say 10–20 minutes. Your sight and sound skills should be your main emphasis as you study for Step 1.

All of you motion learners might be wondering, "What about me?" As a motion learner, you need to think of creating your F.A.C.T.O.I.D. book as part of the "motion"; that is, writing up the wrongs, turning pages during your review, making flashcards, etc. Just as with "muse" learners, you need to develop your sight and sound approaches to learning.

You're going to learn about the AIM YOUR BRAIN Study System and how mixing up the "tags" will help you to avoid boredom and/or feeling overwhelmed. You'll finally be able to take advantage of downtime. You'll be able to reformat the information going in and out of your brain so it will be multiple-choice-question accessible. You'll be studying more skillfully and efficiently as you tune in to your own feats of learning.

CHAPTER 4:

# The AIM YOUR BRAIN®
# Study System

*We aim above the mark to hit the mark.*

— Ralph Waldo Emerson (1803–1882)

## Crossing the Blocked-brain Barrier

As a medical student you know about the blood-brain barrier and its function. Researchers in the early 1900s found:

> ...the brain had a specialized barrier that protected its cells. Dyes injected into the body's blood supply would stain the tissues of most organs—but not the brain. It's now known that a "blood-brain barrier" keeps many substances out of the brain.[20]

I know what you're thinking: *where's she going with this?* Well, even though the body's own blood-brain barrier doesn't really impair the flow of words, key concepts, and future correct answers to multiple-choice exam questions, the metaphor is useful.

Despite the fact that the students I help are highly intelligent, hardworking, and have competitive GPAs, some have difficulty showing what they know on timed multiple-choice

27

examinations. Many just feel like their minds are "clogged up." They truly know the subject matter, but they just can't get it out quickly or accurately enough during the test. So, one day I came up with the idea of a "blocked-brain-barrier" (figuratively speaking) as a way to describe the problem.

**Blocked-brain Barrier:** A condition in which a student knows the subject matter, but just can't get it out quickly and accurately on timed multiple-choice exams.

## How the AIM YOUR BRAIN Study System Came to Be

After working with students for several years, I started to feel that a book like this one might be inside of me. After pharmacy school, but before medical school, I wrote a text-book: *Mathematics For Nurses—With Clinical Applications,* but never a "self-help" book per se. I had kept notes and jotted down ideas, and decided to submit some of my writings to the folks at the Maui Writers Retreat. I was lucky enough to be accepted and get into Sam Horn's "Nonfiction/Self-help" writing group.

Since I didn't know what to expect at the retreat, I just went with the flow. I wrote, turned in my assignments, and active-ly participated in group discussions. During one of the small group sessions, the concept of a "real" system was born. I be-came very excited. It was the first time I had a mental pic-ture that the methods I was using to help my students could even become a system.

Next I realized that I needed to identify the problem: what do students need to do in order to "cross the blocked-brain-barrier"? I felt I was on to something new and that it was a pretty good play on the words of the medical phrase, "crossing the blood-brain barrier." I knew my students would get it and could use it, because that was the whole issue—students trying to get information in and out of their brains in an accessible format, so they could succeed at taking timed multiple-choice tests. The problem was blocked brains, and the solution was a new study system that involved aiming your brain.

The point of the AIM YOUR BRAIN Study System is to transform concepts into little bits of information that can get in and out of your brain quickly and efficiently. In a way it's sort of like sending e-mail messages from your brain—with replies to your brain.

If you're accustomed to reading really dense textbooks and trying to glean important concepts and facts just from reading, you may find yourself falling asleep and not remembering a lot. Unfortunately, when a multiple-choice test is put together, the questions are short paragraphs, cases, or a few lines, with a small selection of answers formatted to test your content recall at a specific moment in time. The AIM YOUR BRAIN Study System is designed to get small bits of information into your "blocked brain" as well as get it out again when you're taking your test.

## The Four-step AIM YOUR BRAIN Study System Revealed

Working with all kinds of students over the years, I've found that many of them have trouble getting newly acquired medical knowledge out of their brains and into the quick-release format needed for timed multiple-choice exams.

I decided to write the AIM YOUR BRAIN Study System in the form of a quatrain, a four-line poem (apologies to Nostradamus and the poetry community). It goes like this:

> ***Do the questions, write the wrongs.***
>
> ***Pursue new Qs all day long.***
>
> ***On F.A.C.T.O.I.D. books, you must depend,***
>
> ***Think you're done? Start again!***

I created these four lines that rhyme (somewhat) to capture the steps needed to study for and pass USMLE Step 1. Think of it as the "AIM YOUR BRAIN quatrain." Each of the four lines represents a single goal. Each will be discussed in detail in the following chapters.

## CHAPTER 5

# Line 1 – Do the Questions, Write the Wrongs

*I approach these questions unwillingly, as they are sore subjects, but no cure can be effected without touching upon and handling them.*

— Titus Livius (59 BC–AD 17)

## Online Question Banks

Feeling overwhelmed is one of the most common problems students encounter when trying to decide what to study to prepare for Step 1. Where do I start? How can I get through everything on the "outline" in the USMLE booklet? Why even bother? Fortunately, there are practice question banks available online that can help focus the content.

I like to look at online question banks as a newer version of an old approach to studying. It used to be that some professors would allow students to use old exams as a means to review for midterms or finals. The student was still expected to attend lectures, turn in homework, and take the quizzes, but the availability of old exams to test your knowledge and simulate your upcoming final was invaluable.

The companies that produce and maintain online question banks provide a service that can help you study more effectively for your online Step 1 exam. As far as I know, none of the companies have inside information on what's going to be on your exam, but they can give you their best estimate of many of the topics and content you might see. If you're wondering whether I have any business connections to any of the online question bank companies, the answer is no!

Working with students preparing for an online exam, I've found that it makes sense to use online practice questions. These can be studied in blocks and timed in a manner similar to the "real" exam. The online question banks keep track of your progress, and your answers and scores are accessible 24/7 (except for occasional website maintenance).

So what makes a good online question bank? You have to have enough questions to practice, but not so many that you'll never get through them. The questions should simulate those found on the real exam. Remember: none of the companies can know exactly what's on the test, but they can design their online question banks as good approximations. The answers and explanations should be well written and not confusing. The website should be user-friendly and simple to navigate. The scoring and tracking methods should be easy to understand. The exams should be able to be timed. There should be no penalty for going through the question bank as many times as you want.

Some of you may be wondering, why emphasize the questions and not just read the textbooks and review books cover to cover? Unfortunately, the reading-only approach doesn't work as well for multiple-choice exams. Reading is passive, and you need active preparation for a multiple-choice exam. That said, if you have extra time you can do your in-depth reading and work the AIM YOUR BRAIN program together. The days of reading textbooks cover to cover and hoping the information gets into your brain are over. In the next section we'll compare a few of the popular online question banks.

## Specific Online Question Banks

My students seem to favor Kaplan's online question bank (however, UsmleWorld.com is becoming more and more popular), and a few still like The Princeton Review and Exam Master®. Since my role is to be the coach, I usually adjust the AIM YOUR BRAIN system to work with whichever online question bank my students choose.

Kaplan's Qbank consists of 2,350 questions and costs $189 (USD) for 3 months. I usually ask my students to work in timed blocks of 50 questions per 60 minutes. If you do 100 questions per day, you'll get through them in 24 days. Two hours of 100 questions (TIMED) will take 1–4 hours to write up, depending on how many you missed; how many notes you write in the F.A.C.T.O.I.D. format; how quickly you can write (legibly); and how much additional information you include from other brief references or notes from previous class lectures.

UsmleWorld.com has been known for its Step 2 preparation, but recently seems to be gaining on Kaplan for Step 1. UsmleWorld.com's online question bank consists of ~ 2,000 questions and costs $185 (USD) for 3 months.

Finally, we are left with The Princeton Review and Exam Master®. You may have other sites that you use, and that's fine. The Princeton Review's online question bank used to consist of 2,000 + questions and costing $149 US for 3 months, but now the website has changed. They seem to be pushing their comprehensive package and not showing a price. Exam Master® has 7,700 questions for $99 (USD) per month for online access. They also have a CD-ROM for $179 (USD). [By the way, I think 7,700 questions are way more than you need to prepare for Step 1 using the AIM YOUR BRAIN® system, but if you're a glutton for punishment, then be my guest.]

Since the number of questions and prices are subject to change, here are the websites for the most up-to-date information:

**www.kaplanmedical.com**; **www.Usmleworld.com**;

**www.princetonreview.com**; and

**www.exammaster.com**.

Just click on the info that pertains to USMLE Step 1.

## Fast Start

I'm sure you may be eager to try some of these ideas. I am including this Fast Start section so you can put the words into action. Please remember that this is just a rough guide on how to get started. If you have all the time in the world to study, then you can do fewer questions. The reality is that once you've tried this technique you'll probably need to do more than 100 questions a day. For now, try not to worry about the pace and just do the fast-start tasks.

### Fast Start Tasks

**Task 1:** Sign up for at least a three-month online question bank.

**Task 2:** Buy a spiral bound single subject notebook and several blue or black pens—this notebook will become your F.A.C.T.O.I.D. book (see chapter 7, page 59: Line 3 – On F.A.C.T.O.I.D. Books You Must Depend).

**Task 3:** Do 25 questions (timed), and write up any that you missed in your spiral-bound notebook in the appropriate format *today*. Ignore your score (see the section Finding Your Rock Bottom in this chapter).

**Task 4:** Each week, increase your daily questions by 25 until you're doing 100 questions per day (timed) and writing up the ones you missed.

**Task 5:** Be sure to read through your F.A.C.T.O.I.D. book(s) at least once or twice a week.

**Task 6:** The goal is to get through the online question bank once as quickly as possible.

## What Do I Do with My Other Reference Materials?

That may seem like a dumb question, but it really isn't. All students want to pass their Step 1 exam the first time they take it. Many of your classmates in the years ahead of you have done just that. It's not unusual for you to take their resource recommendations and go out and buy a stack of content-review books. The most important thing you can do with them is hang on to them and try not to buy a whole bunch more for now.

If you've accumulated tall stacks of review books and are starting to feel guilty because you're not using them all simultaneously, it's time to give them a job and then let go of them in your mind. The "new" function of these content-review books will be "for reference only." Try not to feel that you have to read them cover to cover at this point in your study approach. For the time being, just tell your guilty conscience that these books are available for urgent look-ups.

## Finding Your Rock Bottom

When my students first start working with their online question banks, I ask them to do one set of 25 questions (timed, of course). They are required to ignore the score. Really. Are you wondering why? Because it gives them a chance to get used to the AIM YOUR BRAIN Study System. But more important, it gives them a chance to test the water (or wind) and find their "rock bottom," metaphorically speaking.

In *Staying On Top and Keeping Sand Out of Your Pants,* by Scott Miller (no relation) and his colleagues, the authors talk about how important it is to "never enter the water without first knowing the bottom conditions." Their examples involve the world-famous waves off the north shore of Oahu, Hawaii—the Pipeline. They describe the importance of first checking the bottom conditions at the Pipeline. Although the waves look huge and the water deep to a spectator on the beach, danger lurks below. Surfers about to ride the waves near Sunset Beach are at risk of wiping out (or worse) because a shallow coral reef resides just beneath the surface. It's important to find your rock bottom as well. In our case, the rock bottom isn't a coral reef, but something more subtle—unrecognized areas of content weakness. It's essential that you identify your content strengths and weaknesses now, instead of in the form of a wipeout on test day.

## Identifying Strengths and Weaknesses

When you miss a question, it alerts you that this may be a weak area for you. The good news about knowing your areas of weakness is that you can do something to fix them, before taking the actual exam.

I see knowing your strengths and weaknesses as a win-win situation as long as the timing is right. If you know your weak areas before the exam, and design a solution that's customized to your particular style of learning so you'll remember the correction piece, then you've won.

If you identify your weak areas and do nothing about them, then that's a win-lose (at best). No one can know everything, so we need to work on the things that are difficult for us and use the things that come easy as building blocks. As you expand what you know and fill your brain's database with correct concepts and content, you gradually build your self-confidence and grow your self-esteem.

CHAPTER 6

# Line 2 – Pursue New Qs All Day Long

*See first that the design is wise and just: that ascertained, pursue it resolutely; do not for one repulse forego the purpose that you resolved to effect.*

— William Shakespeare (1564–1616)

## Don't Stop Now!

I hope you're experimenting with your fast-start tasks by now and are beginning to get the hang of writing up your incorrect answers in your F.A.C.T.O.I.D. book. It's important that you pursue new Qs all day long because the long-term goal of the AIM YOUR BRAIN System is for you to get through your online question bank as quickly as possible.

That takes planning and commitment. If you're feeling overwhelmed, try to shake it by taking a short walk, going to the gym, playing Sudoku, or whatever refreshes you, and then come back to your online question bank. Keeping to this schedule exposes you to lots of the kinds of questions you'll find on the real exam.

This system is designed to identify your weaknesses and then give you a chance to do something positive about them.

Start small, 25 questions at a time, increasing eventually to 100 or more per session. Remember: the AIM YOUR BRAIN System is far more productive than staring at your piles of review books and falling asleep while you rest your head on them.

## Finding Your Groove

After you've worked the system for a while, you'll start to find your groove. Believe it or not, some students even have fun doing this. Remember: when you miss a question and write it up, you're actually beginning to plug the holes in your knowledge database. This gives you the opportunity to correct false concepts or incomplete recalls, and, with time, allows you to master content not yet tucked into your brain.

Here's the really good news: If you get all of your questions in a block right the first time through, you're golden, and you don't have to write them up. The not-so-good news is if you miss most of them, you must write them up in your F.A.C.T.O.I.D. book. If you miss a bunch of questions, you can not, I repeat, can not, beat yourself up. Do not despair or make negative judgments about yourself; the AIM YOUR BRAIN Study System will help you fix the problem.

## Sample Schedule

Below is a sample schedule to try that's more detailed than the "Fast Start." It's not carved in stone—if you have plenty of time, you can stretch it out; if you're pressed for time, you'll need to compress the to-do list.

# Week 1

## Day 1

**Task 1:** I hope you've signed up for an online question bank. If you haven't, sign up now. Do 25 questions (timed), and write up any that you missed in your F.A.C.T.O.I.D. book today. Ignore your score (see chapter 7, page 59: Line 3 – On F.A.C.T.O.I.D. Books You Must Depend, and chapter 5, page 36 on finding your rock bottom). Total questions = 25.

## Day 2

**Task 1:** In a.m. do 25 questions (timed), and write up any that you missed in your F.A.C.T.O.I.D. book today. Ignore your score.(See chapter 7, page 59: Line 3 – On F.A.C.T.O.I.D. Books You Must Depend, and chapter 5, page 36 on finding your rock bottom). Total questions = 50.

**Task 2:** In p.m. do 25 questions (timed), and write up any that you missed in your F.A.C.T.O.I.D. book today. Ignore your score.(See chapter 7, page 59: Line 3 – On F.A.C.T.O.I.D. Books You Must Depend, and chapter 5, page 36 on finding your rock bottom). Total questions = 75.

## Day 3

**Task 1:** In a.m. do 25 questions (timed), and write up any that you missed in your F.A.C.T.O.I.D. book today. Ignore your score (see chapter 7, page 59: Line 3 – On F.A.C.T.O.I.D. Books You Must Depend, and chapter 5, page 36 on finding your rock bottom). Total questions = 100.

**Task 2:** Read through your F.A.C.T.O.I.D. book twice today. If you're a "sound" learner, read some or all of it aloud once into a tape recorder or MP3 recorder, and then listen to it (see chapter 3, page 21: Feats of Learning).

## Day 4

**Task 1:** Ramp up! In a.m. do 50 questions (timed), and write up any that you missed in your F.A.C.T.O.I.D. book today. Ignore your score. Total questions = 150.

**Task 2:** In p.m. do 50 questions (timed), and write up any that you missed in your F.A.C.T.O.I.D. book today. Ignore your score. Total questions = 200.

## Day 5

**Task 1:** Keep it up! In a.m. do 50 questions (timed), and write up any that you missed in your F.A.C.T.O.I.D. book today. Ignore your score. Total questions = 250.

**Task 2:** In p.m. do 50 questions (timed), and write up any that you missed in your F.A.C.T.O.I.D. book today. Ignore your score. Total questions = 300.

## Day 6

**Task 1:** Read through your F.A.C.T.O.I.D. book once today. If you're a "sound" learner, read some or all of it aloud once into a tape recorder or MP3 recorder, and then listen to it (see chapter 3, page 21: Feats of Learning).

**Task 2:** Take the afternoon off and have some fun. You've gotten through 300 questions in less than a week. You're creating a customized F.A.C.T.O.I.D. book that's helping you identify and correct your weaknesses. You're rebuilding the database in your brain so you can access F.A.C.T.O.I.D.s quickly. Good job!

## Day 7

**Task 1:** Setup a meeting (in the coming week) with your faculty coach to review your progress. If you don't have a faculty coach, try to find one.

**Task 2:** In a.m. do 50 questions (timed) and wirte up those you missed in your F.A.C.T.O.I.D. book today. Ignore your score. Total questions = 350.

**Task 3:** In p.m.. do 50 questions (timed), and write up those you missed in your F.A.C.T.O.I.D. book today. Ignore your score. Total questions = 400.

# Week 2

## Day 1

**Task 1:** Look at your scores and see if you notice any areas that might need some work. Create a specific test of 50 questions, do it, and write up any that you missed in your F.A.C.T.O.I.D. book. It's okay if you need to add a brief note or two in your F.A.C.T.O.I.D. book to help you remember the problem concept. Total questions = 450.

**Task 2:** In p.m. do 50 questions (timed), and write up any that you missed in your F.A.C.T.O.I.D. book today. If you need to create another test on just a single subject, go ahead and do it. If not, just continue to do mixed questions. Total questions = 500.

## Day 2

**Task 1:** In a.m. do 50 questions (timed), and write up any that you missed in your F.A.C.T.O.I.D. book today. Ignore your score. Total questions = 550.

**Task 2:** Read through your F.A.C.T.O.I.D. book once today. If you're a "sound" learner, read some or all of it aloud once into a tape recorder or MP3 recorder, and then listen to it (see chapter 3, page 21: Feats of Learning).

## Day 3

**Task 1:** In a.m. do 50 questions (timed), and write up any that you missed in your F.A.C.T.O.I.D. book today. Ignore your score. Total questions = 600.

**Task 2:** In p.m. do 50 questions (timed), and write up any that you missed in your F.A.C.T.O.I.D. book today. Ignore your score. Total questions = 650.

## Day 4

**Task 1:** Keep it up! In a.m. do 50 questions (timed), and write up any that you missed in your F.A.C.T.O.I.D. book today. Ignore your score. Total questions = 700.

**Task 2:** In p.m. do 50 questions (timed), and write up any that you missed in your F.A.C.T.O.I.D. book today. Ignore your score. Total questions = 750.

## Day 5

**Task 1:** Keep it up! In a.m. do 50 questions (timed), and write up any that you missed in your F.A.C.T.O.I.D. book today. Ignore your score. Total questions = 800.

**Task 2:** In p.m. do 50 questions (timed), and write up any that you missed in your F.A.C.T.O.I.D. book today. Ignore your score. Total questions = 850.

## Day 6

**Task 1:** Read through your F.A.C.T.O.I.D. book once today. If you're a "sound" learner, read some or all of it aloud once into a tape recorder or MP3 recorder, and then listen to it (see chapter 3, page 21: Feats of Learning).

**Task 2:** Take the afternoon off and have some fun. You've gotten through 850 questions in less than two weeks. You're creating a customized F.A.C.T.O.I.D. book that's helping you identify and correct your weaknesses. You're rebuilding the database in your brain so you can access F.A.C.T.O.I.D.s quickly. Good job!

## Day 7

**Task 1:** Be sure to set up a weekly meeting with your faculty coach to review your progress. If you still don't have a faculty coach, continue trying to find one (see chapter 9, page 79: Finding A Faculty Coach).

**Task 2:** In a.m. do 50 questions (timed), and write up any that you missed in your F.A.C.T.O.I.D. book today. Ignore your score. Total questions = 900.

**Task 3:** In p.m. do 50 questions (timed), and write up any that you missed in your F.A.C.T.O.I.D. book today. Ignore your score. Total questions = 950.

# Week 3

### Day 1

**Task 1:** Look at your scores and see if you continue to notice any areas that might need some work. Create a specific test of 50 questions, do it, and write up any that you missed in your F.A.C.T.O.I.D. book. It's okay if you need to add a brief note or two in your F.A.C.T.O.I.D. book to help you remember the problem concept. Total questions = 1,000.

**Task 2:** In p.m. do 50 questions (timed), and write up any that you missed in your F.A.C.T.O.I.D. book today. If you need to create another test on just a single subject, go ahead and do it. If not, just continue to do mixed questions. Total questions = 1,050.

### Day 2

**Task 1:** In a.m. do 50 questions (timed), and write up any that you missed in your F.A.C.T.O.I.D. book today. Ignore your score. Total questions = 1,100.

**Task 2:** Read through your F.A.C.T.O.I.D. book once today. If you're a "sound" learner, read some or all of it aloud once into a tape recorder or MP3 recorder, and then listen to it (see chapter 3, page 21: Feats of Learning).

## Day 3

**Task 1:** In a.m. do 50 questions (timed), and write up any that you missed in your F.A.C.T.O.I.D. book today. Ignore your score. Total questions = 1,150.

**Task 2:** In p.m. do 50 questions (timed), and write up any that you missed in your F.A.C.T.O.I.D. book today. Ignore your score. Total questions = 1,200.

## Day 4

**Task 1:** Keep it up! In a.m. do 50 questions (timed), and write up any that you missed in your F.A.C.T.O.I.D. book today. Ignore your score. Total questions = 1,250.

**Task 2:** In p.m. do 50 questions (timed), and write up any that you missed in your F.A.C.T.O.I.D. book today. Ignore your score. Total questions = 1,300.

## Day 5

**Task 1:** Keep it up! In a.m. do 50 questions (timed), and write up any that you missed in your F.A.C.T.O.I.D. book today. Ignore your score. Total questions = 1,350.

**Task 2:** In p.m. do 50 questions (timed), and write up any that you missed in your F.A.C.T.O.I.D. book today. Ignore your score. Total questions = 1,400.

## Day 6

**Task 1:** Read through your F.A.C.T.O.I.D. book once today. If you're a "sound" learner, read some or all of it aloud once into a tape recorder or MP3 recorder, and then listen to it (see chapter 3, page 21: Feats of Learning).

**Task 2:** Take the afternoon off and have some fun. You've gotten through 1,400 questions in less than three weeks. You're creating a customized F.A.C.T.O.I.D. book that's helping you identify and correct your weaknesses. You're rebuilding the database in your brain so you can access F.A.C.T.O.I.D.s quickly. Good job!

## Day 7

**Task 1:** Be sure to have a weekly meeting setup with your faculty coach to review your progress. If you still don't have a faculty coach, continue to try to find a "pseudo-coach" (see chapter 9, page 79: Finding A Faculty Coach).

**Task 2:** In a.m. do 50 questions (timed), and write up any that you missed in your F.A.C.T.O.I.D. book today. Ignore your score. Total questions = 1,450.

**Task 3:** In p.m. do 50 questions (timed), and write up any that you missed in your F.A.C.T.O.I.D. book today. Ignore your score. Total questions = 1,500.

# Week 4

## Day 1

**Task 1:** Look at your scores and see if you continue to notice any areas that might need some work. Create a specific test of 50 questions, do it, and write up any that you missed in your F.A.C.T.O.I.D. book. It's okay if you need to add a brief note or two in your F.A.C.T.O.I.D. book to help you remember the problem concept. Total questions = 1,550.

**Task 2:** In p.m. do 50 questions (timed), and write up any that you missed in your F.A.C.T.O.I.D. book today. If you need to create another test on just a single subject, go ahead and do it. If not, just continue to do mixed questions. Total questions = 1,600.

## Day 2

**Task 1:** In a.m. do 50 questions (timed), and write up any that you missed in your F.A.C.T.O.I.D. book today. Ignore your score. Total questions = 1,650.

**Task 2:** Read through your F.A.C.T.O.I.D. book once today. If you're a "sound" learner, read some or all of it aloud once into a tape recorder or MP3 recorder, and then listen to it (see chapter 3, page 21: Feats of Learning).

## Day 3

**Task 1:** In a.m. do 50 questions (timed), and write up any that you missed in your F.A.C.T.O.I.D. book today. Ignore your score. Total questions = 1,700.

**Task 2:** In p.m. do 50 questions (timed), and write up any that you missed in your F.A.C.T.O.I.D. book today. Ignore your score. Total questions = 1,750.

## Day 4

**Task 1:** Keep it up! In a.m. do 50 questions (timed), and write up any that you missed in your F.A.C.T.O.I.D. book today. Ignore your score. Total questions = 1,800.

**Task 2:** In p.m. do 50 questions (timed), and write up any that you missed in your F.A.C.T.O.I.D. book today. Ignore your score. Total questions = 1,850.

## Day 5

**Task 1:** Keep it up! In a.m. do 50 questions (timed), and write up any that you missed in your F.A.C.T.O.I.D. book today. Ignore your score. Total questions = 1,900.

**Task 2:** In p.m. do 50 questions (timed), and write up any that you missed in your F.A.C.T.O.I.D. book today. Ignore your score. Total questions = 1,950.

## Day 6

**Task 1:** Read through your F.A.C.T.O.I.D. book once today. If you're a "sound" learner, read some or all of it aloud once into a tape recorder or MP3 recorder, and then listen to it (see chapter 3, page 21: Feats of Learning).

**Task 2:** Take the afternoon off and have some fun. You've gotten through 1,950 questions in less than four weeks. You're creating a customized F.A.C.T.O.I.D. book that's helping you identify and correct your weaknesses. You're rebuilding the database in your brain so you can access F.A.C.T.O.I.D.s quickly. Good job! Depending on which online question bank you're using, you're close to completing one pass through the whole thing.

## Day 7

**Task 1:** Be sure to have a weekly meeting setup with your faculty coach to review your progress. If you still don't have a faculty coach, continue trying to find a "pseudo-coach" (see chapter 9, page 79: Finding A Faculty Coach).

**Task 2:** In a.m. do 50 questions (timed), and write up any that you missed in your F.A.C.T.O.I.D. book today. Ignore your score. Total questions = 2,000.

**Task 3:** In p.m. do 50 questions (timed), and write up any that you missed in your F.A.C.T.O.I.D. book today. Ignore your score. Total questions = 2,050.

# Week 5

### Day 1

**Task 1:** Look at your scores and see if you continue to notice any areas that might need some work. Create a specific test of 50 questions, do it, and write up any that you missed in your F.A.C.T.O.I.D. book. It's okay if you need to add a brief note or two in your F.A.C.T.O.I.D. book to help you remember the problem concept. Total questions = 2,100.

**Task 2:** In p.m. do 50 questions (timed), and write up any that you missed in your F.A.C.T.O.I.D. book today. If you need to create another test on just a single subject, go ahead and do it. If not, just continue to do mixed questions. Total questions = 2,150.

### Day 2

**Task 1:** In a.m. do 50 questions (timed), and write up any that you missed in your F.A.C.T.O.I.D. book today. Ignore your score. Total questions = 2,200.

**Task 2:** Read through your F.A.C.T.O.I.D. book once today. If you're a "sound" learner, read some or all of it aloud once into a tape recorder or MP3 recorder, and then listen to it (see chapter 3, page 21: Feats of Learning).

## Day 3

**Task 1:** In a.m. do 50 questions (timed), and write up any that you missed in your F.A.C.T.O.I.D. book today. Ignore your score. Total questions = 2,250.

**Task 2:** In p.m. do 50 questions (timed), and write up any that you missed in your F.A.C.T.O.I.D. book today. Ignore your score. Total questions = 2,300.

## Day 4

**Task 1:** Keep it up! In a.m. do 50 questions (timed), and write up any that you missed in your F.A.C.T.O.I.D. book today. Ignore your score. Total questions = 2,350.

**Task 2:** Take the afternoon off—you deserve it!

## Day 5

**Task 1:** Read through your F.A.C.T.O.I.D. book once today. If you're a "sound" learner, read some or all of it aloud once into a tape recorder or MP3 recorder, and then listen to it (see chapter 3, page 21: Feats of Learning).

**Task 2:** Read chapter 8: Line 4 — Think You're Done? Start Again! Don't panic. This will be the best part.

## Day 6

**Task 1:** Be sure to set up a weekly meeting with your designated faculty coach or pseudo-coach to review your progress.

**Task 2:** Start doing the questions in your online question bank again (second pass through). In a.m. do 50–75 questions (timed), and write up any that you missed in your F.A.C.T.O.I.D. book today. Watch your score go up. You'll have fewer to write up in your F.A.C.T.O.I.D. book. Questions = 50 min/75 max.

**Task 3:** In p.m. do 50–75 questions (timed), and write up any that you missed in your F.A.C.T.O.I.D. book today. Questions = 100 min/150 max. The number of minimum and maximum questions per day is just an estimate.

## Day 7

**Task 1:** Take a whole day off.

# Week 6

## Day 1

**Task 1:** Look at your scores and watch them go up. Do 50–100 questions (timed), and write up any that you missed in your F.A.C.T.O.I.D. book. It's okay if you need to add a brief note or two in your F.A.C.T.O.I.D. book to help you remember the problem concept. Questions = 150 min/250 max.

**Task 2:** In p.m. do 50–100 questions (timed), and write up any that you missed in your F.A.C.T.O.I.D. book today. Questions = 200 min/350 max.

## Day 2

**Task 1:** In a.m. do 50–100 questions (timed), and write up any that you missed in your F.A.C.T.O.I.D. book today. Questions = 250 min/450 max.

**Task 2:** Read through your F.A.C.T.O.I.D. book once today. If you're a "sound" learner, read only the new F.A.C.T.O.I.D.s aloud once into a tape recorder or MP3 recorder, and then listen to all of your recordings once (see chapter 3, page 21: Feats of Learning).

## Day 3

**Task 1:** In a.m. do 50–100 questions (timed), and write up any that you missed in your F.A.C.T.O.I.D. book today. Ignore your score. Questions = 300 min/550 max.

**Task 2:** In p.m. do 50–100 questions (timed), and write up any that you missed in your F.A.C.T.O.I.D. book today. Savor your score. Questions = 350 min/650 max.

## Day 4

**Task 1:** Keep it up! In a.m. do 50–100 questions (timed), and write up any that you missed in your F.A.C.T.O.I.D. book today. Ignore your score. Questions = 400 min/750 max.

**Task 2:** In p.m. do 50 questions (timed), and write up any that you missed in your F.A.C.T.O.I.D. book today. Questions = 400 min/750 max.

## Day 5

**Task 1:** Keep it up! In a.m. do 50–100 questions (timed), and write up any that you missed in your F.A.C.T.O.I.D. book today. Questions = 550 min/850 max.

**Task 2:** Take the afternoon off—you deserve it!

## Day 6

**Task 1:** Read through your F.A.C.T.O.I.D. book once today. If you're a "sound" learner, read only the new F.A.C.T.O.I.D.s aloud once into a tape recorder or MP3 recorder, and then listen to all of your recordings once (see chapter 3, page 21: Feats of Learning).

**Task 2:** In p.m. do 50–100 questions (timed), and write up any that you missed in your F.A.C.T.O.I.D. book today. Questions = 600 min/950 max.

## Day 7

**Task 1:** Meet with your designated faculty coach or pseudo-coach on a weekly basis.

**Task 2:** In a.m. do 50–100 questions (timed), and write up any that you missed in your F.A.C.T.O.I.D. book today. Watch your score go up. You'll have fewer to write up in your F.A.C.T.O.I.D. book. Questions = 650 min/1,050 max.

**Task 3:** In p.m. do 50–100 questions (timed), and write up any that you missed in your F.A.C.T.O.I.D. book today. Ignore your score. Questions = 700 min/1,150 max.

# Week 7

## Day 1

**Task 1:** Look at your scores and watch them go up. Do 50–100 questions, and write up those you missed in your F.A.C.T.O.I.D. book. It's okay if you need to add a brief note or two in your F.A.C.T.O.I.D. book to help you remember the problem concept. Questions = 750 min/1,250 max.

**Task 2:** In p.m. do 50–100 questions (timed), and write up those you missed in your F.A.C.T.O.I.D. book today. Questions = 800 min/1,350 max.

## Day 2

**Task 1:** In a.m. do 50–100 questions (timed), and write up any that you missed in your F.A.C.T.O.I.D. book today. Questions = 850 min/1450 max.

**Task 2:** Read through your F.A.C.T.O.I.D. book once today. If you're a "sound" learner, read only the new F.A.C.T.O.I.D.s aloud once into a tape recorder or MP3 recorder, and then listen to all of your recordings once (see chapter 3, page 21: Feats of Learning).

## Day 3

**Task 1:** In a.m. do 50–100 questions (timed), and write up any that you missed in your F.A.C.T.O.I.D. book today. Ignore your score. Questions = 900 min/1,550 max.

**Task 2:** In p.m. do 50–100 questions (timed), and write up any that you missed in your F.A.C.T.O.I.D. book today. Savor your score. Questions = 950 min/1,650 max.

## Day 4

**Task 1:** Keep it up! In a.m. do 50–100 questions (timed), and write up any that you missed in your F.A.C.T.O.I.D. book today. Ignore your score. Questions = 1,000 min / 1,750 max.

**Task 2:** In p.m. do 50 questions (timed), and write up any that you missed in your F.A.C.T.O.I.D. book today. Questions = 1,050 min / 1,850 max.

## Day 5

**Task 1:** Keep it up! In a.m. do 50–100 questions (timed), and write up any that you missed in your F.A.C.T.O.I.D. book today. Questions = 1,200 min / 1,950 max.

**Task 2:** Take the afternoon off—you deserve it!

## Day 6

**Task 1:** Read through your F.A.C.T.O.I.D. book once today. If you're a "sound" learner, read only the new F.A.C.T.O.I.D.s aloud once into a tape recorder or MP3 recorder, and then listen to all of your recordings once (see chapter 3, page 21: Feats of Learning).

**Task 2:** In p.m. do 50–100 questions (timed), and write up any that you missed in your F.A.C.T.O.I.D. book today. Questions = 1,250 min / 2,050 max.

## Day 7

**Task 1:** Have your weekly meeting with your designated faculty coach or pseudo-coach.

**Task 2:** In a.m. do 75-150 questions (timed), and write up any that you missed in your F.A.C.T.O.I.D. book today. Watch your score go up. You'll have fewer to write up in your F.A.C.T.O.I.D. book. Questions = 1,325 min/2,200 max.

**Task 3:** In p.m. do 75-150 questions (timed), and write up any that you missed in your F.A.C.T.O.I.D. book today. Ignore your score. Questions = 1,400 min/2,350 max.

## In The Remaining Time

Go through your F.A.C.T.O.I.D. book a few more times. If you're still having difficulty with a specific concept, then get out your "reference" books and write up a few notes in your F.A.C.T.O.I.D. book.

Obviously, the more questions you can do per day the faster the whole process goes. If you use an online question bank with fewer questions, you'll get through it sooner.

It's also important to remember that if you're on a rotation or in class all day, you'll have to modify your study schedule and still find time to do your online questions.

If you're lucky enough to have a day or two off, you'll need to ramp up the number of questions you do per day to make up for the days when you couldn't get to them.

CHAPTER 7

# Line 3 – On F.A.C.T.O.I.D.® Books You Must Depend

*Real, constructive mental power lies in the creative thought that shapes your destiny, and your hour-by-hour mental conduct produces power for change in your life. Develop a train of thought on which to ride. The nobility of your life as well as your happiness depends upon the direction in which that train of thought is going.*

— Laurence J. Peter (1919–1988)

## Definition of F.A.C.T.O.I.D.

According to *Webster's New World Dictionary and Thesaurus*, the word "factoid" means "a single fact or statistic variously regarded as being trivial, useless, unsubstantiated, etc." Although many of you may feel that the multiple-choice exam questions you've seen in the past, which seemed to be based on minutia, fit the literal definition of factoid, the way we're going to use the word is as an acronym. For this book, the abbreviation F.A.C.T.O.I.D. means "Frequently Asked Concepts To Own In Depth."

Stay with me here. Multiple-choice questions are nothing more than inquiries about how much you know about a subject and how well you understand key concepts. The idea behind F.A.C.T.O.I.D.s is that you are actively learning and remembering little facts that are short and to the point so they can readily pass into and out of your brain. By breaking down complex information into shorter sentences or phrases, you're able to handle the key concepts more efficiently. By having small bits, or "bytes," of information go in and out of your brain, you're better prepared to recall and recognize specific F.A.C.T.O.I.D.s during your timed multiple-choice exams.

The AIM YOUR BRAIN Study System is designed to expose you to important "frequently asked concepts" so that you know them and can recall them quickly and easily. If you really know a key concept then it's yours to own. Content books give you references that you can use for review. The AIM YOUR BRAIN System makes sure that you convert your weak areas into concepts that you can store accurately in your brain's database for rapid future retrieval.

## How to Make a F.A.C.T.O.I.D. Book

As you may recall, in the fast-start section in chapter 5, you were told to go to the store and buy a few items if you didn't already have them. For those of you who skipped the fast-start and mock-schedule sections, here's what you need to do:

- Buy several spiral-bound single subject notebooks. Do not get one of those five-subject doodads (if this sounds a little authoritarian, I apologize — at least you get to choose the color of your F.A.C.T.O.I.D. book cover.)

- Ditch the highlighters and use one color of ink, black or blue.

- Make sure there's lots of white space: one line of space between similar concepts, two lines of space between new concepts.

## F.A.C.T.O.I.D. Format Examples

Let's take another look at the sample questions from chapter 2. Each of the three examples is in a multiple-choice format and contains a stem, distracters, and the correct answer. In real life, if you miss any of the questions while using your online question bank, you have an opportunity to review an explanation of the correct answer.

To make the sample questions more real, I've added an explanation to each of the three examples. Please take a moment to review the three sample questions, answers, and explanation.

## Example 1

A twenty-two-year-old woman has just been diagnosed with HIV. She has heard about a new class of medications called integrase inhibitors. Which of the following drugs is an integrase inhibitor? [STEM]

(A) Lamivudine        [DISTRACTER]

(B) Raltegravir       [CORRECT ANSWER]

(C) Ribavirin         [DISTRACTER]

(D) Rifampin          [DISTRACTER]

(E) Ritonovir         [DISTRACTER]

## Explanation

There are currently six classes of antiretroviral drugs. The following table lists them individually.[21] Multi-class combination products are listed as well. Raltegravir is the first integrase inhibitor (AKA HIV integrase strand transfer inhibitor) currently available. Lamivudine (3TC) is a nucleoside reverse transcriptase inhibitor (NRTI). Ribavirin is an antiviral nucleoside analogue used in combination with interferon to treat hepatitis C. Rifampin is an antimycobacterial agent commonly used to treat tuberculosis (TB). Ritonovir (RTV) is a protease inhibitor (PI).

## Drugs Used in the Treatment of HIV Infection

| *Multi-class Combination Products* | | | | |
|---|---|---|---|---|
| **Brand Name** | **Generic Names** | **Manufacturer Name** | **Approval Date** | **Time to Approval** |
| Atripla | efavirenz, emtricitabine and tenofovir disoproxil fumarate | Bristol-Myers Squibb and Gilead Sciences | 12-July-06 | 2.5 months |

| *Nonnucleoside Reverse Transcriptase Inhibitors (NRTIs)* | | | | |
|---|---|---|---|---|
| **Brand Name** | **Generic Name(s)** | **Manufacturer Name** | **Approval Date** | **Time to Approval** |
| Combivir | lamivudine and zidovudine | GlaxoSmithKline | 27-Sep-97 | 3.9 months |
| Emtriva | emtricitabine, FTC | Gilead Sciences | 02-Jul-03 | 10 months |
| Epivir | lamivudine, 3TC | GlaxoSmithKline | 17-Nov-95 | 4.4 months |
| Epzicom | abacavir and lamivudine | GlaxoSmithKline | 02-Aug-04 | 10 months |
| Hivid | zalcitabine, dideoxycytidine, ddC | Hoffmann-La Roche | 19-Jun-92 | 7.6 months |
| Retrovir | zidovudine, azidothymidine, AZT, ZDV | GlaxoSmithKline | 19-Mar-87 | 3.5 months |
| Trizivir | abacavir, zidovudine, and lamivudine | GlaxoSmithKline | 14-Nov-00 | 10.9 months |
| Truvada | tenofovir disoproxil fumarate and emtricitabine | Gilead Sciences, Inc. | 02-Aug-04 | 5 months |

| Brand Name | Generic Name(s) | Manufacturer Name | Approval Date | Time to Approval |
|---|---|---|---|---|
| Videx EC | enteric coated didanosine, ddl EC | Bristol Myers-Squibb | 31-Oct-00 | 9 months |
| Videx | didanosine, dideoxyinosine, ddl | Bristol Myers-Squibb | 9-Oct-91 | 6 months |
| Viread | tenofovir disoproxil fumarate, TDF | Gilead | 26-Oct-01 | 5.9 months |
| Zerit | stavudine, d4T | Bristol Myers-Squibb | 24-Jun-94 | 5.9 months |
| Ziagen | abacavir sulfate, ABC | GlaxoSmithKline | 17-Dec-98 | 5.8 months |

### (NNRTIs)

| Brand Name | Generic Name | Manufacturer Name | Approval Date | Time to Approval |
|---|---|---|---|---|
| Intelence | etravirine | Tibotec Therapeutics | 18-Jan-08 | 6 months |
| Rescriptor | delavirdine, DLV | Pfizer | 4-Apr-97 | 8.7 months |
| Sustiva | efavirenz, EFV | Bristol Myers-Squibb | 17-Sep-98 | 3.2 months |
| Viramune | nevirapine, NVP | Boehringer Ingelheim | 21-Jun-96 | 3.9 months |

### Protease Inhibitors (PIs)

| Brand Name | Generic Name(s) | Manufacturer Name | Approval Date | Time to Approval |
|---|---|---|---|---|
| Agenerase | amprenavir, APV | GlaxoSmithKline | 15-Apr-99 | 6 months |
| Aptivus | tipranavir, TPV | Boehringer Ingelheim | 22-Jun-05 | 6 months |
| Crixivan | indinavir, IDV | Merck | 13-Mar-96 | 1.4 months |
| Fortovase | saquinavir (no longer marketed) | Hoffmann-La Roche | 7-Nov-97 | 5.9 months |
| Invirase | saquinavir mesylate, SQV | Hoffmann-La Roche | 6-Dec-95 | 3.2 months |
| Kaletra | lopinavir and ritonavir, LPV/RTV | Abbott Laboratories | 15-Sep-00 | 3.5 months |
| Lexiva | Fosamprenavir Calcium, FOS-APV | GlaxoSmithKline | 20-Oct-03 | 10 months |
| Norvir | ritonavir, RTV | Abbott Laboratories | 1-Mar-96 | 2.3 months |
| Prezista | darunavir | Tibotec, Inc. | 23-Jun-06 | 6 months |
| Reyataz | atazanavir sulfate, ATV | Bristol-Myers Squibb | 20-Jun-03 | 6 months |
| Viracept | nelfinavir mesylate, NFV | Agouron Pharmaceuticals | 14-Mar-97 | 2.6 months |

| Fusion Inhibitors | | | | |
|---|---|---|---|---|
| Brand Name | Generic Name | Manufacturer Name | Approval Date | Time to Approval |
| Fuzeon | enfuvirtide, T-20 | Hoffmann-La Roche & Trimeris | 13-Mar-03 | 6 months |

| Entry Inhibitors - CCR5 co-receptor antagonist | | | | |
|---|---|---|---|---|
| Brand Name | Generic Names | Manufacturer Name | Approval Date | Time to Approval |
| Selzentry | maraviroc | Pfizer | 06-Aug-07 | 8 months |

| HIV integrase strand transfer inhibitors | | | | |
|---|---|---|---|---|
| Brand Name | Generic Names | Manufacturer Name | Approval Date | Time to Approval |
| Isentress | raltegravir | Merck & Co., Inc. | 12-Oct-07 | 6 months |

At this point it's important to make a few notes in your F.A.C.T.O.I.D. book (see fig. 7–1) that will help you remember the information. If you missed the question, you must correct your misinformation now and jot down a few brief notes so you won't miss the question again. The notes you write can be in outline form or as single sentences. On occasion you may end up photocopying a chart or graph you have from previous lectures or readings and pasting or taping it into your F.A.C.T.O.I.D. book. That's fine, just don't spend all your time putting together a "scrapbook" and not getting through your questions for that day. Remember to include lots of white space between your entries. Also please don't copy the entire question, answer, and explanation word for word from your online question bank. I don't want you to break any copyright rules. The pages in your F.A.C.T.O.I.D. book might look like the following (see fig. 7–1 and 7–2):

6 classes of AntiRetroViral (ARV) drug classes for HIV/AIDS

– Nucleoside Reverse Transcriptase Inhibitors (NRTIs)

   – – Lamivudine

– Nonnucleoside Reverse Transcriptase Inhibitors (NNRTIs)

– Protease Inhibitors (PIs)

   – – Ritonovir

– Entry Inhibitors – CCR5 co-receptor antagonists

–HIV Integrase strand transfer inhibitors

   – – Raltegravir

Fig. 7–1. New F.A.C.T.O.I.D. book page

*Ribavirin = antiviral nucleoside analogue used in combination with interferon to treat hepatitis C.*


*Rifampin = antimycobacterial agent commonly used to treat tuberculosis (TB).*

Fig. 7–2. Continuation of F.A.C.T.O.I.D.
book notes on new page

The white space makes it easier to review your F.A.C.T.O.I.D. book in future. If you cram all your F.A.C.T.O.I.D.s so tightly onto a few pages that you can't read them, you've wasted your time. If you don't include white space, and the F.A.C.T.O.I.D. book pages are covered with a dense forest of ink, you won't want to use it as much. Your eyes see "too much to read" and your brain thinks "too much to review." Having some white space enables you to add other notes and information. Many textbooks are trying to engage the brain with white space, color, and images. Your customized F.A.C.T.O.I.D. book will engage your brain as well; give it a chance.

## Example 2

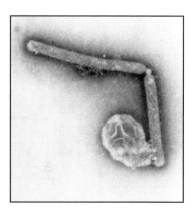

**Fig. 2.1:
Influenza A *virions*.**[9]

During August to October 2004, sporadic human cases of bird flu were reported in Vietnam and Thailand. The above transmission electron micrograph (TEM) shows two of the avian influenza A virions. What is the influenza A virus sub-type of greatest concern for avian flu?

    (A) H1N1        [DISTRACTER]

    (B) H1N2        [DISTRACTER]

    (C) H3N2        [DISTRACTER]

    (D) H4N1        [DISTRACTER]

    (E) H5N1        [CORRECT ANSWER]

### Explanation

There are three types of influenza viruses: A, B, and C. Only influenza A viruses are further classified by subtype on the basis of two main surface glycoproteins: hemagglutinin (HA) and neuraminidase (NA).[22] Subtypes of influenza A that are currently circulating among people worldwide include H1N1, H1N2, and H3N2 viruses. Influenza viruses are normally highly species-specific. Since 1959, instances of human infection with an avian influenza virus have been documented on only 10 occasions. Of the hundreds of strains of avian influenza A viruses, only four are known to have caused human infections: H5N1, H7N3, H7N7, and H9N2. The H5N1 virus is highly pathogenic. Of all influenza viruses that circulate in birds, H5N1 is of greatest present concern for human health.[23] H4N1 is not a current subtype.

Take a look at Fig. 7–3 and notice how it is growing. The entries are a little closer together than in Fig. 7–1. This is really personal preference. The main point is spreading things out and lots of white space.

*Ribavirin = antiviral nucleoside analogue used in combination with interferon to treat hepatitus C.*

*Rifampin = antimycobacterial agent commonly used to treat tuberculosis (TB).*

*3 Types of Influenza Viruses*
  *–A*
  *–B*
  *–C*

*Subtype classification*
  *– Only pertains to influenza A*
  *– Based on surface glycoproteins*
  *– – hemagglutinin (HA)*
  *– – neuraminidase (NA)*

*4 subtypes of influenza A caused by human infections*
  *–H5N1 = greatest concern, highly pathogenic*
  *– H7N3*
  *– H7N7*
  *– H9N2*

*Other subtypes circulating in humans*
  *– H1N1*
  *– H1N2*
  *– H3N2*

Fig. 7–3. F.A.C.T.O.I.D. book page with less white space

Please observe that I just continued writing my notes where I left off from the last entry. Don't try to organize your notes by topic. Your F.A.C.T.O.I.D. book entries are somewhat random, and that keeps things interesting.

## Example 3

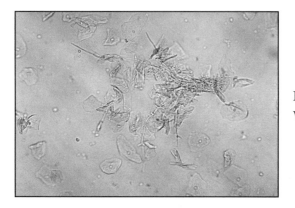

Fig. 2.2: Vaginal wet mount.[10]

The above wet mount shows what type of infection?

(A) **Bacterial vaginosis**          **[DISTRACTER]**

(B) *Candida Albicans*          **[CORRECT ANSWER]**

(C) *Chlamydia trachomatis*          **[DISTRACTER]**

(D) *E. coli*          **[DISTRACTER]**

(E) *Trichomonas vaginalis*          **[DISTRACTER]**

## Explanation

The three diseases most frequently associated with vaginal discharge are: bacterial vaginosis (BV—replacement of normal vaginal flora by an overgrowth of anaerobic microorganisms, i.e., *Gardnerella vaginalis*); trichomoniasis (*T. vaginalis*); and candidiasis (usually caused by *Candida albicans*). Discharge can be further examined by diluting one sample in one to two drops of 0.9% normal saline solution on one slide and a second sample in 10% potassium hydroxide (KOH) solution. An amine odor detected immediately after applying KOH suggests BV. Cover slips are placed on the slides, and they are examined under a microscope at low-and high-dry power. Motile *T. vaginalis* or clue cells (epithelial cells with borders obscured by small bacteria), which are characteristic of BV, usually are identified easily in the saline specimen. The yeast or pseudohyphae of Candida species are more easily identified in the KOH specimen.[24] The slide pictured above shows a yeast infection caused by *Candida albicans*. *E. coli* and Chlamydia infections are usually not diagnosed by wet mount (see Fig.7–4 for F.A.C.T.O.I.D. book page notes).

*3 most common diseases with vaginal d/c*

*- Bacterial vaginosis (BV)*
*-- overgrowth of anerobes*
*-- Gardnerella vaginalis*
*-- amine odor with KOH*
*-- clue cells*

*- Trichomoniasis*
*-- T. vaginalis*
*-- motile on saline specimen*

*- Candidiasis*
*-- usually caused by Candida albicans*
*-- pseudohyphae with KOH*

*- Wet mount*
*-- 1-2 drops of NS on one slide*
*-- few drops of 10% KOH on second slide*
*-- cover slides*
*-- microscopy @ low-dry and high-dry power*

Fig. 7–4: F.A.C.T.O.I.D. book page continuation

I've just started a new page. When you write up your next question, just skip a few lines and keep going. If the above looks too dense to you, then skip a line between each thing you write. There's no wrong way to do this as long as you include a reasonable amount of white space.

## Using Your F.A.C.T.O.I.D. Books for Review

Okay, now that you have this lovely creation called a F.A.C.T.O.I.D. book, you may be wondering how to use it. I'm glad you asked.

Since the notes you put into it are determined by what questions you missed, you're going to use your F.A.C.T.O.I.D. book to understand the things you didn't know well enough in the beginning.

F.A.C.T.O.I.D. books should be reviewed once or twice a week. This may seem like a lot, but it gets easier as you do it. If you're still going through online question banks and writing up the questions you missed, no problem—just pick a few times a week and review what you have in one, two, or more F.A.C.T.O.I.D. books.

If you get tired of reviewing your F.A.C.T.O.I.D. books silently, how 'bout an audio version? You can use a cassette recorder, MP3 recorder, or PC, and make audio versions by just reading aloud. You might ask, "And just why would I want to do this?" Simple—it's useful. You can listen to yourself speak while you're commuting to class or the hospital, during a run or workout, or whenever. It's efficient use of otherwise downtime. It helps keep your learning active and fresh. It mixes things up and helps keep you from getting bored.

Many of my students find that reviewing their F.A.C.T.O.I.D. book(s) frequently helps to cement concepts. If all goes well, eventually you'll see your notes in your brain, even visualizing your handwriting on individual pages.

Your F.A.C.T.O.I.D. books are powerful because they represent areas of prior weakness in your knowledge base that you have corrected and mastered. If you think about it, that's quite an accomplishment.

It's important to know that your F.A.C.T.O.I.D. books should not be shared. They are uniquely you and are in a way bonded to your brain. It's *your* eyes seeing *your* notes in *your* handwriting or hearing *your* voice on *your* audio reviews. Since you paid for an online service that's registered to you, you need to be respectful of copyright law and keep notes on the questions you missed, and additional notes from your readings and classroom work, to yourself. Of course, if you have questions, you can share your F.A.C.T.O.I.D. books with your faculty coach for clarification and guidance.

CHAPTER 8

# Line 4 – Think You're Done? Start Again!

*Vitality shows in not only the ability to persist
but the ability to start over.*

— F. Scott Fitzgerald (1896–1940)

## *Groundhog Day* Replay? Not!

In the movie *Groundhog Day,* Bill Murray plays Phil Con-
nors, a TV weatherman who is asked for the fifth year in a
row to cover the Groundhog Day celebration in Punxsutaw-
ney, Pennsylvania. He doesn't want to do it and can hardly
wait to finish the assignment—but this year something weird
happens after the celebration. A severe winter storm knocks
out phone service and closes the roads. When Phil wakes up
the next morning, and every morning after that, he discov-
ers it's February 2, Groundhog Day, all over, again and again.
He's caught in what seems to be an endless time loop.

First, let me reassure you that you're not going to be caught
in an endless online question-bank loop. Repeating the online question bank over and over again may seem like déjà
vu (you know—the feeling that you've done this before),
but it's an extremely important step. By redoing the online

question bank, you get to experience repetition and build your self-confidence.

The first time through, you were exposed to a huge collection of content in a multiple-choice question format. When you repeat the process with the same questions, you're storing in your mind the concepts you'll need for easy future access.

You might be wondering how completing the first three steps of the AIM YOUR BRAIN Study System (AKA the first three verses of the "AIM YOUR BRAIN Quatrain") helps you now. That's easy. The first three steps have provided you with:

- A targeted review;

- An active learning approach;

- The realization that there is light at the end of the tunnel;

- A means to achieve peak performance on test day.

## Savor Your Accomplishments So Far

So what have you really accomplished so far? You've gotten through your online question bank once. That's great, it's a huge thing. You have a composite score based on "mixed" questions. (Don't panic). You've created a F.A.C.T.O.I.D. book or books that you've been reviewing by reading silently, reading aloud, or listening to portions in your car or while exercising, etc. Your F.A.C.T.O.I.D. book represents previous weaknesses that you've corrected or are close to correcting. Pretty good, huh?

## How To Start Again

Now the fun starts. It's time to go back through the online question bank and continue to do blocks of questions. Rest assured, this time the questions will go quicker because you've seen them before.

If you miss any questions the second time through, then you need to write them up (even if you've written them up before). If you need to add an additional concept or note from other sources, do it now and do it quickly.

You'll start seeing your individual test scores go up. Check the test analysis section of your online question bank. As your scores go up, so does your confidence.

At some point you'll start to recall information you learned in the classroom; now you have it in a format that's useful during timed multiple-choice exams. When you get to this point in the study system, you may find yourself with a funny grin on your face (it's okay to smile and feel good about your achievements). You're heading toward mastering concepts that were already in your brain. You just needed to find a way to get them into a format that's useful for the dreaded standardized testing that we all have to go through.

## CHAPTER 9

# Finding A Faculty Coach

*The best advisers, helpers and friends, always are not those
who tell us how to act in special cases, but who give us, out of
themselves, the ardent spirit and desire to act right, and leave
us then, even through many blunders, to find out what our
own form of right action is.*

— Phillips Brooks (1835–1893)

## What's A Faculty Coach, and Why Do I Need One?

A faculty coach is usually a member of your medical school's full-time basic science or clinical faculty or a volunteer faculty member. This person should be someone with whom you feel comfortable, someone you can talk to easily, someone you can trust to guide you, and someone to whom you will be accountable.

Performance accountability is the main reason you need a faculty coach. When you work alone, it's very easy to blow off your AIM YOUR BRAIN Study System assignments. Your faculty coach can help you do something that's difficult to do alone.

Sometimes when you're in the middle of a huge project — and yes, preparing for you Step 1 exam is a huge project — it's helpful to have another person around to help you do the things that are tough to do alone. Your faculty coach can help you define your weak areas and honestly introduce correction pieces when necessary. Your faculty coach can provide the support and guidance you need, as well as review your scores, assign the number questions per day each week, and help you plan your overall strategy for tackling Step 1 using the AIM YOUR BRAIN Study System.

## How Do I Find My Own Faculty Coach?

The way to start is by asking yourself: who has a reputation as someone who helps students? Remember: the people to consider are usually your basic science faculty, clinical faculty, and volunteer faculty. Depending on how your medical school's curriculum is organized you may know quite a few clinical faculty or you may not. Many medical schools are introducing clinical experiences before the third year, or students may be introduced to clinical faculty via their longitudinal patient-case coursework, etc.

Another question you need to ask when searching for your prospective faculty coach: Whom do others regard as a "real "teacher"? Those faculty members who enjoy teaching and helping students usually have some if not all of the following characteristics: they possess excellent communication skills and knowledge of their area of expertise, are fair-minded, are perceived by others as student advocates, radiate warmth and trust, and are excited about learning new things in their daily life.

You're probably wondering where to look for this amazing

faculty coach. The answer is usually pretty easy—ask around: You can ask your advisor, ask your friends, ask your upper classmates, or ask your ombudsperson (if your school has one). Also, depending on how things are going, you might not have a choice, i.e., your school's Student Progress Committee or Performance Committee or equivalent may refer you.

If, after all of the above, you still haven't found a real faculty coach, then it's time for a substitute. Ask someone you trust and who you think can be neutral to step in as your "pseudo-faculty" coach. The candidates are usually friends or family members. The problem is that these relationships usually carry a lot of baggage — whether the baggage is good or bad is irrelevant.

With a friend or family member in the role of pseudo-faculty coach, you're at risk of falling back into old relationship routines and roles that you gave up a long time ago: times when you got help with homework from Mom and Dad; imposed on friends who were busy with their own careers; or asked your spouse or significant other to become your taskmaster instead of your source of comfort and support. I'm not saying it can't work. It can, but it's just harder. My advice is: if you've asked a faculty member and he or she said no, keep looking.

## A Little Homework Never Hurt Anyone

One thing we need to get straight right off the bat: you're going to have homework—no ifs, ands, or buts! Homework is an integral part of active learning. Remember: in the AIM YOUR BRAIN Study System you need to work with targeted content. You're using multiple-choice question content to lead you to mastery of multiple-choice exam concepts.

You will be doing the following types of fun-filled homework:

- Timed-question blocks;

- Missed-question write-ups;

- F.A.C.T.O.I.D. notebook reviews.

In addition, you may find yourself listening to audio CDs, tapes, or MP3 files, using flash cards, or reviewing favorite charts, graphs, or notes from you classroom work to fill in the areas you still need to work on.

## "You've Got Mail." Weekly Progress Meetings and E-mail Updates

Every time I meet my students face to face, they leave with one of my "green sheets." There's nothing special about the "green sheets" per se; they're plain 3 × 4-inch tablets with my name, department, and phone number. I started using them because they were handy and plentiful.

As I meet with each student, I take notes on the green sheet, list goals, and create tasks aimed at achieving those goals. After our session I make a copy of the green sheet for myself and give my student the original. (Please note the "green sheet" pictured is white, not green. Use your imagination.)

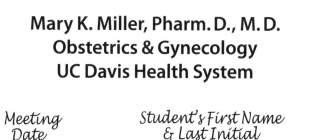

**Mary K. Miller, Pharm. D., M. D.**
**Obstetrics & Gynecology**
**UC Davis Health System**

| Meeting Date | Student's First Name & Last Initial |
|---|---|

☐ Sign up for online question bank

☐ Buy single-subject spiral notebook

☐ Use either blue or black pen

☐ You get to pick notebook cover

☐ Start with 25 questions— timed

☐ Write up the wrongs in your F.A.C.T.O.I.D. book as instructed

☐ MKM mtg next week Date and Time

The best way to monitor your progress is via weekly face-to-face meetings with your coach; the second best is via email, and third best is via phone calls. I think face-to-face meetings are the best because they give both of you the opportunity to build the relationship.

You need a faculty coach who's familiar with the way you think, react, and deal with the ups and downs of Step 1 preparation. There have been times when my students have needed additional support due to a family crisis or to unexpected responses from residents, faculty, and classmates; and because of our coaching relationship, I was able to help more effectively. Sometimes I do coach a student intermittently via e-mail or phone, but my preference is in person.

Weekly face-to-face meetings work best if both you and your faculty coach are punctual. My students know that if I meet them after clinic, I may be late depending on how well the residents, patients, and I can keep to the schedule. In this case, my students just bring something to study, knowing that I'll get to my office as soon as possible. If you or your faculty coach have some unexpected conflict and can't meet, be sure to call, page, or e-mail each other as soon as you know. If possible, don't wait till the last minute.

Our flexible agenda usually consists of:

- **Check-in (how did the previous week go?);**
- **F.A.C.T.O.I.D.notebook review;**
- **Look at online question scores together;**
- **New task assignments for the coming week.**

It's important that you and your faculty coach have a way to measure your progress. To do this your faculty coach needs to be able to monitor your online progress. You need to respect the website's rules and regulations, so it's probably best to log on to the website during a face-to-face meeting so you can briefly show your results to your faculty coach in person.

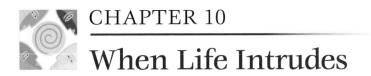

# CHAPTER 10

# When Life Intrudes

*Life can only be understood backwards;*
*but it must be lived forwards.*

— Soren Kierkegaard (1813–1855)

## Finding Time to Study
## When There Is None

Life is full of interruptions. Unfortunately, being a medical student doesn't protect you from these occurrences. Your workload in your preclinical years increases dramatically. There's never enough time to do everything, and finding the time to study for Step 1 when there is none can be quite challenging. The bottom line is you have to make a plan that includes unplanned interruptions and you have to stick to it.

In *Eat That Frog!* author Brian Tracy discusses how to get important things done fast. The title of his book is based on words attributed to Mark Twain: "If you eat a frog first thing in the morning, the rest of your day will be wonderful."[25] What he's really saying is that if you organize your day and tackle your most important task first, then you'll feel a greater satisfaction and sense of accomplishment.

In case you haven't figured it out yet, USMLE Step 1 is your "frog." The first thing you need to do to tackle this task is to plan and set your priorities wisely. The best way to devise a study plan is to get a timer, set it for 15 minutes, then take a sheet of paper and make a list of everything on your mind right now. When the timer goes off, take a breather and see how you feel. Everything cluttering your mind is now on paper. In a few minutes you'll be resetting your priorities and you'll be on your way to finding time to study when there is none. Let's take a closer look at procrastination, which is one of the biggest reasons why there never seems to be enough time.

> **Procrastination is defined as "to put off doing something, especially out of habitual carelessness or laziness"; also, "to postpone or delay needlessly."** [26]

Obviously some procrastination is good, and some is bad. We need to know the difference between the two kinds and then be able to do something about the bad. None of us can do everything that needs to get done. You will end up postponing something, but it's vital that you put off only less important activities and do the hardest task first. In your case, it's going to be getting through the assigned number of questions in your online question bank, writing up the wrongs in your F.A.C.T.O.I.D. book(s), and reviewing your F.A.C.T.O.I.D. book(s), etc.

> **self‑dis • ci • pline**: Training and control of oneself and one's conduct, usually for personal improvement. [27]

The most obvious thing that can be said about the term self-discipline is that it has something to do with change and hard work. Self-discipline sounds like an old-fashioned concept, and it may be, but a lot of people have achieved their goals because of it. I surmise that your determination and hard work got you into medical school, even though the application process, interviews, and waiting for an acceptance letter may seem so long ago.

I include the definition of self-discipline in this chapter because you're going to need it when life intrudes—and it will. Preparing for your Step 1 exam will be hard work. Why? Because putting off studying for it until the last minute is the usual modus operandi. "I'm too busy to study for Step 1, I have final exams coming up"; "I do great on standardized exams, I always wait till the last minute"; and, in the words of that great philosopher Alfred E. Newman, "What, me worry?" (*MAD* magazine, 1955).

If you don't view the USMLE Step 1 exam as challenging, and you blow off the hard work it will take to pass it, then you should be worried. This is where the ideas from *Eat That Frog* come in. When you do the work in a disciplined way, you lay the foundation for studying for future multiple-choice examinations that will come into your life over and over again. Remember what Brian Tracy, author of *Eat That Frog,* says: "Persistence is actually self-discipline in action." Be persistent in keeping to your goal of being well prepared for Step 1. Now we'll look at workload considerations and how to study effectively.

You've probably discovered by now that medical school is completely different from your undergraduate experience. In medical school you sit in lecture halls with the same 100 to 120-plus classmates. You may be in smaller group settings as well, but for the most part you're linked to the same classmates for most of your first two years.

The workload is heavier, and the time you need to spend studying after class and on weekends can be all consuming, and you have lots and lots of tests. Just when you think you've earned a break in the form of a little time off, you start feeling guilty and find yourself hitting the books again. Then, just before your third year starts, you have to take USMLE Step 1.

When you start to prepare for Step 1 your workload changes: You still need to keep up with your courses, but now you have to find time to study for the USMLE as well. You may find yourself more isolated and wondering how to change gears for Step 1.

That's what this book is for. If you start early enough, you can run through the Step 1 online questions as you study for your class exams — *and* you can write up the wrongs and use your new F.A.C.T.O.I.D. book as review tool for both exams.

Some students find study groups helpful after they've been studying for Step 1 for a while. The increased workload is not going away, so success in medical school is all about finding a way to handle it. Success in studying for Step 1 is starting early.

Interruptions aren't going away as you study for your boards. You need to be able to carve out some uninterrupted time to achieve your daily study goals. Perhaps the best way to do this is to make a repeating appointment with yourself and let those around you know that you're unavailable except in case of an extreme emergency.

Set specific times and find a quiet place where you can work without interruption. If you go to the library, consider getting one of those little glassed-in rooms, and face away from the door if possible. If you're at home, go to your desk area and put a sign on the door that lets people know you're un-available. If you're a parent, your spouse will have to keep the little one(s) occupied elsewhere. The key is to have a predefined start and finish time; when you're done, you can return calls and do all the things that didn't get done while you were studying for your Step 1 exam. If your friends or family are helping by running interference for you, be sure to find ways to return the favor after your exam.

If you're "studying" at the local coffee or tea hangout, once again you have to try to position yourself so you're away from the action. Wear headphones (even if you're not listen-ing to music) and try not to make eye contact with everyone who passes by. You are there to study and pass your Step 1 exam. Lattes are okay.

One way of avoiding interruptions is to make sure you're sending out the right DON'T INTERRUPT ME NOW cues: Close your door if you can; silence your cell phone; disable or show busy on your instant messager and chats. If you're busy writing in your F.A.C.T.O.I.D. book or hammering away at your keyboard, then the message is clear to most people— I'm busy!

It's important to look at the problem of interruptions because they're real, and they won't go away without some kind of intervention on your part. The real problem with interrup-tions is the cost to the work you're doing currently. If you're just signing onto your online question bank or reviewing a few pages in your F.A.C.T.O.I.D. book, then you can start and stop easily. If, however, you're in the middle of a timed on-line test, or you finally just figured out why you keep miss-ing the same question over and over again and you need to make some quick notes, you might not be able to get back to the same "zone" after being interrupted.

## Saying No to Family and Friends

One of the hardest things you may have to do while studying for USMLE Step 1 is say no to family and friends. Everyone knows that medical school can be all consuming, but till now we've tried to find a balance between class work and home life. Since many of you aren't in formal Step 1 preparation classes, you must carve out the time to study using whatever free minutes and hours are left.

This is really the process of setting boundaries in your life. You can't do everything, and you absolutely have to focus on preparing for your Step 1 exam. It's crucial that you take the time to study now, and pay back the time to your family and friends later. I'm not saying you should become a hermit for several months and pop back into your former life the minute you walk out of the test center, but you may have to make some difficult choices. Some likely examples:

- Not being able to go on the entire weeklong family vacation (if possible, go for a few days instead).

- Not being able to see every one of your son's or daughter's soccer games (try to get to one or two; get a copy of the schedule and commit to those that are doable).

- Not being able to spend the weekend in the city with your old college roommates (take a rain check or commit to Saturday night only and leave early Sunday morning).

Sometimes you will cause hurt feelings. I wish it weren't so, but it is. Unless you're married to or dating another medical student who's going through or has recently gone through what you're experiencing, it's possible your significant other (SO) will have a hard time understanding—most people just can't. For better or worse, the process of becoming a physician is grueling and at times the obstacles can feel insurmountable. Even if your significant other's heart is in the right place, the medical school process can change you both.

In time, most of us find our "old" selves again, and reclaim the part of us that we had to push aside for a while. Your loved ones will change as well, and they'll forgive you for the things you did, the hurt feelings you caused, and the things you missed out on.

Remember: You've worked really hard to get to this place in your medical career. Your family and friends are proud of you and want you to succeed. If you have to say no, remember to emphasize that it's temporary, and schedule something to do with them after the exam.

It's important to have a plan for those people who aren't in your inner circle, such as friends and relatives who live out of town. If they call and say they'd like to drop in for a stay, direct them to the nearest reasonably priced motel and meet them for dinner or breakfast. If you have a significant other (spouse, partner, etc.), he or she will probably be the one running interference for you. Remember to plan something really special for your SO after this is all over.

If you find yourself listening to insensitive remarks from other people who think they understand what you're going through but don't have a clue—"it's only a test," "when I took it twenty years ago, I barely had to study for it," etc.,—walk away quickly. You don't need to hear it and you don't need to deal with it. Forget about it!

Also remember: You're not alone. If you need to talk to your classmates about strategies for carving out time, do it. Just don't take too much time.

## Escape to Your Third Place

Traditionally speaking, the concept of a "third place" is meant to represent a place other than your home or work space. Ray Oldenburg, creator of the term, explains in his book, *The Great Good Place,* that third places are simply "informal public gathering places."[28] His concept revolves around the idea that people need informal public places to gather and interact, such as coffee shops and general stores, so they can get to know each other and have a sense of community.

In medical school, the library or quad area may become a third place, and in the spirit of *The Great Good Place,* these may work fairly well, but I have a definition for "third place" that's different from Mr. Oldenburg's. My meaning has to do with finding a place of solitude, not comradeship. The first time I heard the term "third place" was at the Maui Writer's Retreat. My writing mentor, Sam Horn, told our group about the concept as it pertains to writers.

Writers have a process that helps them put pen to paper (in my case font to screen). Many can write at home after everyone else goes to bed, and some can get up before dawn and write. Others, such as J. K. Rowling of Harry Potter fame, went to her favorite coffee shop and wrote away. I can write in the morning, but I don't have enough time. It seems I just get into it and it's time to get ready for work. I tried Starbucks and Java City, but I dislike having to pick up my laptop and take it into the restroom so it won't get stolen.

Writing at work doesn't do it for me either. As the clinic medical director and teaching attending, there's just too much going on. I've found that leaving the house and going to a small apartment works best for me. I can write for a few days, go home and spend time with my family and friends, and then be ready for work on Monday. It might sound extravagant, but it's what I need to do to think and write.

My students have had to find their own third place, a place where they can get away from the demands of home and school or work, a place where they know they can study without interruptions. Some students work in the library. Others pick a coffee shop or cafe that's somewhat noisy. They tell me they know that not all test centers are quiet, and they want to get used to the background noises of people pointing and clicking and typing away. Your third place is wherever works best for you.

Some students can study at home or in their apartment. Like Stephen King, they have created a third place in their first place. In his book *On Writing,* King talks about how he created his writing room in his own home. He also stresses the importance of "working in a serene atmosphere."[29]

As much as my soul agrees with Professor Oldenburg's concept of a third place as somewhere that people can gather and share stories, we must not go there when it's time to study for Step 1. It's vital that you find a third place that's more like a writer's refuge to focus on your Step 1 preparation. When it's time for a break, go find one of Oldenburg's "great good places" and share conversation and community with all your heart.

## Crisis Management 101

There is a great Web resource that deals with students and crisis management. It's a Peace Corps Resource adaptation by SAFETI (Safety Abroad First Educational Travel Information) found at www.globaled.us.

No one really talks about crisis management and the USMLE, but I've seen students thrown into chaos during unexpected events. Some of my students have had to deal with family members' illnesses and deaths, feelings of helplessness and worry as friends and families face disasters half a world away, the death of a classmate, or the sudden breakup of a committed relationship.

We can't plan for everything, but it's helpful to have a general approach to certain types of crises. Most of the crises my students have experienced are of a more personal nature rather than regional, national, or international. The main theme has been family medical emergency.

As noted in the SAFETI resource, most crises have several things in common:

- They can result in a disruption or early termination of study.

- They usually cause significant emotional stress, resulting in predictable cognitive, physical, and behavioral reactions.

- They can be managed with the appropriate support and preparation.

If a crisis occurs, try to remain calm. In most cases, as the identified medical student, your family and your friends who aren't in med school already see you as the one who "knows what to do." Even if you're not sure, put your training, experience, and insight into action. If a relative has collapsed, be sure to perform your basic life support and have someone call 911 (or emergency services). It's amazing how many families are afraid to call for help. If one of your grandparents has died unexpectedly, your family and friends may look to you for answers. If your child or spouse is injured, you're expected to fix it or do the right thing.

Then, in the aftermath of crisis, you're expected to keep studying and take your exam as scheduled, essentially pretending that nothing out of the ordinary has happened. In actuality, things have changed, you have changed, and you need to talk it over with your faculty coach.

I've seen my students reluctant to mention anything about a family crisis, because they didn't want to get off target with their study plan. As their faculty coach, I've helped them make the hard decisions: take a few days off to be at the hospital with family; postpone the exam; and/or notify the appropriate authorities at the Dean's Office or Student Affairs.

Remember: A true crisis can happen to anyone. It's important to try to plan as best you can, even if it's something as basic as remaining calm and getting help. Talk to your faculty coach so he or she can help you figure out a solution and find any additional resources (psychological, administrative, etc.), you might need. With appropriate support and a little preparation, most crises can be managed—even those that interfere with USMLE Step 1 preparation.

# CHAPTER 11

# Conquering Test Anxiety

*Any fact facing us is not as important as our attitude toward it, for that determines our success or failure. The way you think about a fact may defeat you before you ever do anything about it. You are overcome by the fact because you think you are.*

— Norman Vincent Peale (1898–1993)

## Test Anxiety-A-Little-Bit

Test anxiety as defined by Spielberger and Vagg (not to be confused with Spielberg of *Jurassic Park* fame) can be thought of as a situation-specific anxiety trait that involves the frequency and intensity of the emotional reactions and worry cognitions that students experience during examinations.[30]

Nearly all of us have experienced test anxiety sometime in our lives. If you haven't, then you're lucky. When you felt the test anxiety coming on, most likely you were either able to work through it and finish the exam with a decent score, or you found yourself going blank and unable to retrieve the information you studied prior to the test. Next you started to worry about finishing the remaining questions correctly and within the time limit. Probably, self-doubt crept into your mind, and your score was just barely passing or worse.

If any of this sounds familiar, read on and learn what you need to do to conquer test anxiety.

Among my favorite sessions during my OB/GYN residency were the interactive pathology sessions given by Dr. Richard Oi. He had a great way of describing things. He was not only an obstetrician and gynecologist, but a pathologist as well. When he talked about cervical intraepithelial neoplasia, CIN 1, CIN 2, and CIN 3, he would draw a diagram that represented a cervical biopsy with a progressive increase in the number of abnormal cells. The histology with just a small amount of abnormal cells was "CIN-a-little-bit," and the ones with almost all abnormal cells (but with an intact basement membrane, of course) was "CIN-Lotsa." So I'm borrowing Dr. Oi's descriptors: test anxiety that's mostly mild will be called Test Anxiety-a-little-bit, and moderate to debilitating test anxiety will be called Test Anxiety-Lotsa.

As you know by now, medical school can be very stressful, and having to take an endless number of exams can worsen that stress. Test anxiety is a form of stress that flares up when you have to take a test, and when it comes to multiple-choice exams, the anxiety some students feel can be overwhelming. For some "otherwise capable medical students… performance anxiety so debilitating as to compromise their performance on professional licensing examinations."[31]

I've had students with differing degrees of test anxiety, ranging from minimal to incapacitating. No matter where you see yourself on this continuum, it's a topic worthy of discussion, because there are things you can do to help yourself. Some techniques and treatments are easier than others.

## Test Anxiety-Lotsa

There are many components to debilitating test anxiety (DTA). The simplest definition that captures the essence of the problem is from Professor Albert Bandura's book *Self-Efficacy:* "Anxiety is defined as a state of anticipatory apprehension over possible deleterious happenings."[32] The best definition I've found as it applies to USMLE type exams is "Severe anxiety symptoms occur in anticipation of and/or during professional licensing examinations, particularly those that contain test questions in a multiple-choice format. These examinations produce disabling worry, emotionality, and autonomic hyperarousal."[31]

Almost everyone on the planet has experienced some kind of nervousness before they perform. If you sing, dance, read poetry, play an instrument, engage in competitive athletics, speak in front of an audience, or take oral or multiple-choice exams, you've felt it: butterflies in your stomach as you wait for your onstage cue; the adrenaline rush as you race out of the starting blocks on the track, hoping to qualify for the team; the doubt that creeps into mind as you wait for the proctors to give you the signal to begin your exam. We wish we could turn off this part of our sympathetic nervous system, but it's the same process we need to stay alert and focused throughout any challenge. There has to be a happy medium, and usually, most of us can find it.

Unfortunately, not everyone can control their test anxiety, no matter how hard they try. This is where the techniques and sometimes treatment come into play. Moderate to debilitating test anxiety can cause the "dual deficits" of poor test preparation, poor test performance, or both.[31]

## Techniques to Quell Test Anxiety-A-Little-Bit

There are all kinds of breathing exercises to help you relax and calm down. If you have a favorite, practice it before the exam to make sure it's working for you. One approach I like is the 5-5-5 × 5:

1. While sitting up in your chair, close your eyes.

2. Inhale through your nose to a silent count of 5 and hold it for another count of 5.

3. Slowly exhale through your mouth while silently counting to 5 once more.

4. Concentrate only on your breathing, and nothing more.

5. Repeat the whole inhalation-exhalation process a minimum of 5 times.

6. If you get dizzy, stop immediately—you're probably blowing off too much $CO_2$.

One of the most helpful techniques I share with my students is visualization. I ask them to visualize a special place they can go to in their minds to help center themselves. To explain, I tell them that my place is snorkeling in the ocean on the Kohala Coast of the Big Island of Hawaii. I can see beautiful fish and coral and sunbeams slanting down through the crystal-clear water, and sea turtles swimming toward the surface. It's very quiet, just the occasional sound of water lapping gently on the nearby rocks as I float to the surface and look back at the beach.

Once I share my place, they get the idea and usually come up with one of their own. If they need a little help, I usually ask a series of questions and together we can find their place.

Once the place is set in their minds, I ask them to practice going there as they study. I urge them to do this several times before our next scheduled meeting. I also ask them to go there if they start feeling anxious about the test. We practice this at subsequent meetings. I often have them use this technique as I describe the following scenario: "You're at the test center and you've started your computerized exam. As you look over the first six or seven questions, you start to panic because you can't remember the information you need to answer any of those questions."

I have them go to their place in their mind for a few moments, and then they're usually able to go on, first answering the questions they know, and, when less stressed, returning to the ones that almost stopped them cold. Our running joke is that it's okay to go to your place in your mind, but you can't stay there for more than a few moments—if you get so relaxed and calm that you doze off, you've been there too long.

The best way to deal with negative thoughts is to stop them immediately and replace them with positive self-talk. If the negative thoughts are invading your mind, you need to take aggressive action.

- **In your mind, say, *STOP* or *NO*.**

- **Immediately start telling yourself, "I can do this"; "I really know my stuff"; "This time *is* different"; or whatever you can come up with.**

- **If you're having trouble with this, talk to your faculty coach right away.**

When a play or musical is about to open, the cast and crew go through dress rehearsals to work out the bugs and make any last-minute changes. It's important that you perform a "test rehearsal" in your mind before you ever step into the test center. The key to making this work for you is to deliberately cause the anxiety in your mind and then use the above techniques to deal with it. So here we go:

Imagine it's the night before your exam, and you're worried about tomorrow. As you start to feel anxious, you need to intervene:

- Say NO or STOP to any negative thoughts.

- Replace any negative thoughts with positive self-talk.

- Do your 5-5-5 × 5 breathing exercise.

- Go to your place in your mind and center yourself.

- Use any or all of the above in any order.

- Take a break.

Substitute a different scenario and practice reducing your anxiety:

- You've driven to the test center and can't find a parking place.

- You're at your computer in the test center and it malfunctions.

- You've looked at the first five questions on the screen and you don't know the answer to any of them.

- You look at your watch, you have only ten minutes left, and you still have twenty questions to go.

Create your own scary scenario and then intervene.

## Test Anxiety-Lotsa Treatment

If you think you might have Test Anxiety-Lotsa, it's time to see a psychologist. There's only so much your faculty coach can do, and then it's time for the expert. If I can give you just one piece of advice, it's do it now and not later.

Some of my students have had debilitating test anxiety (DTA). I've been able to offer emotional support and improve their test preparation by teaching them the AIM YOUR BRAIN Study System, but I don't have the skills to treat their DTA. I've helped them find someone who could see them privately and protect their confidentiality. I know this is a huge step, but you need to take it as soon as possible. The sooner you get professional help the better you'll feel.

If you have an underlying depression or generalized anxiety disorder, then medication may need to be prescribed by a psychiatrist adept at pharmacotherapy. If you have DTA only, then medications don't usually work that well. Behavioral therapy is usually superior to medication, because the drugs may dull your ability to work though your anxiety. "Exposure-based treatment can eliminate anxiety. Use of benzodiazepines to target and reduce anxiety is the polar opposite of the exposure, which is aimed at evoking anxiety in order to extinguish it and pave the way for the new learning of effective coping."[33] Exposure therapy is similar to the test-rehearsal technique, but in greater depth.

Most students are reluctant to seek treatment. I can't emphasize this enough: if you have moderate to debilitating test anxiety you need to "suck it up" and go see a psychologist. Remember: If major athletes can get help from a psychologist to improve their game, then we should be able to as well. They'll say it's a performance issue, and that's partly true, but it's actually a performance anxiety disorder. An estimated 2% of the US population is afflicted by debilitating performance anxiety.[34] Guess what? Debilitating test anxiety is also a performance anxiety disorder — and it's treatable.

## CHAPTER 12

# Set the Stage for Your Success

*Courage and perseverance have a magical talisman, before which difficulties disappear and obstacles vanish into air.*

— John Quincy Adams (1767–1848)

## The End Is In Sight

I'm sure you're wondering what John Quincy Adams's quote on courage and perseverance has to do with setting the stage for your success (and what the heck does the word "talisman" mean?). I know what you're thinking: here's another old saying and a definition for a word that most people have never heard before. Indulge me for just a moment.

John Quincy Adams's words are profound. One definition for talisman is "anything whose presence exercises a remarkable or powerful influence on human feeling or actions."[35] Combined with this, Adams's meaning becomes "Courage and perseverance have a magical and powerful influence on human feeling or actions, before which difficulties disappear and obstacles vanish into air." Not bad, huh? That's the essence of this chapter. Courage, perseverance, and let's not forget, a little planning. You're almost done with all of this preparation; the end is in sight.

## Courage

It takes courage to change your life around so that you can carve out the time needed to study for USMLE Step 1. It takes courage to find a faculty coach to help you. It takes courage to go through your online question bank a second time, not fully believing your test scores will go up enough (but they will). It takes courage to show up at the test center and sit for your Step 1 examination. It takes courage to continue working through the test blocks when you're distracted by the law student sitting next to you, loudly hammering away at the keyboard as he takes the bar exam. It takes courage not to walk out the door during a break because you don't think you're doing well. It takes courage to suppress your test anxiety when you see the first exam questions on your computer screen. It takes courage to see a psychologist or psychiatrist to help you with your debilitating test anxiety.

Remember, courage is "the quality of mind or spirit that enables a person to face difficulty, danger, pain, etc., without fear; bravery."[36] You have already shown great courage in this endeavor.

## Perseverance

According to dictionary.com the term "perseverance" means "steady persistence in a course of action, a purpose, a state, etc., esp. in spite of difficulties, obstacles, or discouragement."[37]

You've worked hard to reach this point. You've worked diligently, following the AIM YOUR BRAIN Study System. You've created your F.A.C.T.O.I.D. book(s), and reviewed them until you can't look at them anymore. You've taken those content areas that gave you trouble in the past and you now own them. You have overcome the obstacles. You have truly persevered. You haven't given up, and you are ready to face Step 1.

## A Little Planning Goes A Long Way

Before giving a formal talk, I visit the room where I'll be speaking, ahead of time. If the schedule permits, I go the night before or early in the morning. I check out which side the podium sits on, and look around to see if there are any obstructions to the screens. I bring my own laptop as a backup, as well a copy of the presentation on some kind of portable medium. Why do I do this? Because it makes me feel better and more confident. In *What's Your Point,* Bob Boylan's book on making presentations, he talks about the importance of being prepared and how that responsibility is yours. "Speakers don't use Murphy's Laws—they use O'Toole's. Murphy said: 'If anything can go wrong it will.' O'Toole said: 'Murphy was an optimist'."[38] In addition, Boylan says: "The presenter has the final responsibility for the room." [38]

I believe when you go to take your Step 1 examination, you have the responsibility to familiarize yourself with the test site beforehand. Just as I take the time to know my presentation site, you must know your test site. You need to find the time to:

1. Make a test run to the center a day or two before your scheduled exam.

2. Check out the parking situation.

3. Know the public transportation routes and schedules and be sure they are running on time.

4. Have money for a taxi as a backup plan.

5. Be sure you know the location of the restrooms.

6. Get the weather forecast; bring a raincoat, umbrella, etc., if it looks like rain, and bundle up if it's going to snow.

If you're spending the night at your own apartment or residence, then your surroundings are more familiar. Be sure to practice your techniques for minimizing test anxiety. If you get anxious, work through it yourself or phone your faculty coach or your psychologist. This is not the time to call up classmates who share your situation; they're probably anxious, and you don't need to be around other anxious people. Also, the night before your test, don't call up classmates who've already taken the exam. They may inadvertently say the wrong thing and set you off inside. Stay centered and focused on you.

If you're staying at a motel, hotel, or any unfamiliar place, try to make it more homelike. Bring something familiar from home—a photo, clock, or special object, and set it where you can see it. If you're staying only one night and checking out the next morning, then make sure your belongings are safe and secure. If you need to store your luggage at the hotel, just do it.

## Test-day Packing List

Be sure to bring:

1. Scheduling permit

2. Acceptable picture ID, such as your

  a. Driver's license with photo of you

b. Passport

c. National Identity Card

d. Other government-issued ID that's still in-date

e. ECFMG-issued ID card

3. Snacks (for breaks)

4. Water, beverages (for breaks)

5. Soft earplugs

6. The outfit you plan to wear (lay it out the night before).

7. MP3 player with earphones and a play list of music that calms or inspires you (you can listen to it if you feel stressed before the exam).

8. Please see your current USMLE Bulletin for specific rules at testing sites.

## "Centered" Exam Strategies

It is now time to apply your techniques and remain calm and focused. Take a moment to imagine a meeting between you and your faculty coach on the day before your exam. I'll play the role of your coach, and you... you can be yourself. The dialogue might go something like this:

**STUDENT**: "You know, the test is tomorrow."

**COACH:** "Yes, that's why I'm glad we're meeting. I wanted to check in and see how you're doing."

**STUDENT:** "I'm glad we're meeting, too. I feel ready, but I'm a little nervous."

**COACH:** "Nervousness the day before the exam is normal. I do have a few things I'd like to go over again, okay?"

**STUDENT:** "Okay."

**MKM:** "These are the things I want you to remember. I want you to get a good night's sleep tonight. I want you to make sure you have all your things, all the food and other stuff you're going to bring with you. And I want to make sure that you're okay emotionally during the exam."

**STUDENT:** "What should I do if I go blank?"

**COACH:** "The chances of that happening are really remote, but let's say you open the test, the screen comes up, you look at it, and you go, 'Oh no, where did these questions come from? I don't know any of this. I'm going home,' that's when I want you to take a few deep breaths. I want you to visualize your special place in your mind, the place that we've worked out, and center yourself. And then keep moving. It's okay if you don't know an answer. Mark the ones you don't know. You *will* come to those questions where you do know the answer, so just jump right back in and go for it. Later, go back to the ones that you marked and do them."

**STUDENT:** "What if I don't know the answer for sure?"

**COACH:** "Then you'll have to make an educated guess. Remember what F.A.C.T.O.I.D. means: 'frequently asked concepts to own in-depth.' By now you own your F.A.C.T.O.I.D.s. They may throw some things at you that you don't know, but that's okay. Be confident in knowing what you *do* know. After reading the question carefully, if you can get rid of three of the distracters because you know they aren't true, then you have a 50/50 chance of getting it right."

**STUDENT:** "Okay. Do you think I'll have enough time to finish?"

**COACH:** "Yup. Remember: as you worked through your online question bank, you did it timed. Right?"

**STUDENT:** "Yes, that's right."

**COACH:** "Well, your pace was actually about a minute a question. That pace should continue to work for you. And since we are talking about time, remember to take a couple of five-minute breaks partway through (after block 2 and 3 if you need to) before your lunch break. During lunch, take no more than thirty minutes to eat and refresh. Then re-center yourself and keep moving."

**STUDENT:** "Knowing me, sometimes during long tests I just want to get through it quickly and leave."

**COACH:** "If you start having these thoughts, you need to say *STOP!* in your mind, and take a moment to regroup. You know the importance of perseverance (I didn't write it to use up ink and cut down trees). Remember the definition: 'steady persistence in a course of action… in spite of difficulties, obstacles, or discouragement.' You have the tools to get through this exam as planned. Use them. If you still have time, take a break."

**STUDENT:** "I will. Thanks for taking the time to help me. I really appreciate it. I'll let you know how tomorrow goes."

**COACH:** "I'm happy to help. Remember: you can do this!"

You can't control everything. Try to be prepared for anything and have a strategy to deal with surprises, i.e., computer glitches, no earplugs allowed at your center, etc. Expect the unexpected calmly. Remember: you, too, can do this!

## The Waiting Game

The current minimum passing score on USMLE Step 1 using the three-digit scale is 185 (two-digit scale is 75). Remember: the passing score is reviewed periodically and can be changed, so before you take your exam it's important to take a look at the USMLE website, www.Usmle.org, and keep the minimum passing score in mind.

The test scores are released each week on Wednesdays. The range for your exam is somewhere between three and six weeks from the time you took your test. Most students get their scores within three to four weeks. The results are now available online by logging onto your registration entity website, NBME or ECFMG.

> *Between the wish and the thing life lies waiting.*
>
> — Anonymous

Once the test is over, do your exam post-mortem and get on with your life. Try to use the anxiety-reducing techniques in chapter 11 to help with the waiting.

You deserve a few rewards after all your hard work. Here are a some suggestions.

1. Sleep in.

2. Do something fun—go skiing, go to the beach, go for a long hike in the hills.

3. Reconnect with your family and friends.

4. Choose your own special reward.

It's important to pull out your positive self-talk to help you while you wait. Sometimes it's hard to do the same things you did prior to your exam. A positive affirmation tape, CD, or MP3 audio presentation may be helpful. I like Wayne Dyer's *Meditations for Manifesting: Morning and Evening Meditations to Literally Create Your Heart's Desire* (especially the morning ones, but any will do). If you have a spiritual, meditative, or religious practice that you prefer, then use it.

In closing, it's important for you to reflect on and understand that you have given this exam your best shot. I'm proud of the work you've done, and I wish you all the success in the world. Thank you for choosing to spend some of your valuable time with me via this book.

# APPENDIX 1

## Brief History of the NBME/USMLE

## NBME History

As promised in chapter 1, the rest of the NBME history is included here. So what really happened?

In the late 1800s, individual states were licensing their own doctors and there was very little reciprocity between them. What really triggered the change toward a national licensing concept started with one man, Dr. William Rodman. Dr. Rodman lived in Kentucky. He had been asked to be the chair of surgery at the Medico-Chirurgical College in Philadelphia, Pennsylvania. He had already passed his Kentucky licensing boards, but still had to go up and take the Pennsylvania boards.[1] He wasn't too happy about this.

In the years that followed, Dr. Rodman lobbied for the idea of setting up a National Board of Medical Examiners that would provide a uniform method of licensure. He was the president of the Association of American Medical Colleges (AAMC) and the American Medical Association (AMA) during his career. By 1915, the National Board of Medical Examiners was formed; it still exists today. Not bad for the inspiration and hard work of one guy.

## USMLE History

The USMLE Step series has morphed from the original week-long, (yes, I said weeklong) written, oral, and clinical endurance questioning, to the essay, written, and practical oral examinations at the bedside.

Prior to the USMLE, US allopathic medical students usually took either the NBME (Parts I, II, and III) or the FLEX (Component 1 and 2) examinations. Beginning in 1992, the USMLE became the single examination for medical licensure in the United States.

Today the three-part written and the one-part clinical skills exams are sponsored by the Federation of State Medical Boards (FSMB) and the National Board of Medical Examiners (NBME).

## Money, Money, Money

You know better than anyone that taking USMLE Step 1 is a costly proposition. The examination fee is approaching $500 US each time. When you add the cost of buying review books, online question banks, etc. it all adds up. I feel that it's important to keep this money thing in perspective. No matter how the national licensing exam started (remember 1915), it's now big business for the NBME. Based on a 2004 Form 990 from the IRS, the revenue for examination fees from individual applicants was over $50 million. My point? They make more money if you fail. Try to be well prepared ahead of time, and practice, practice, practice your techniques to remain calm, centered, and focused. Keep your money for yourself.

# APPENDIX 2

# Exam Do-overs

## No Pinocchio Noses Here

The children's story *Pinocchio* was originally written by the Italian writer Carlo Lorenzini, under his pen name Carlo Collodi. It was first published in 1881. The main character, Pinocchio, was a wooden puppet boy, carved by the poor carpenter Geppetto. Pinocchio came to life and had many adventures and life lessons to learn. Pinocchio's most famous attribute was that whenever he told a lie, his nose grew longer.

Not passing USMLE Step 1 can be a devastating experience. After the initial shock wears off, fear, loss of self-esteem, and sometimes shame usually remain. You may know exactly what went wrong or you may not. At some point you'll have to answer one question truthfully: "how much did I really study?"

This is the time for soul searching and brutal honesty with yourself. If you didn't put in the time for effective, focused study, then admit it now, and accept it. If you have moderate to debilitating test anxiety, admit it now, and accept it. If you have a suspected or diagnosed learning disability, admit it now, and accept it. If something else is going on, figure it out, admit it now, and accept it.

To pass Step 1, a new plan based on a factual evaluation of your previous study methods is vital. There can't be any Pinocchio noses in your self-assessment of the situation.

## "I Did It My Way."
## A Hard Look at Test Preparation

### *Effective vs. Ineffectual Approaches*

The key word here is "insight." Do you have any real clue what went right and what went wrong? Take a look at the following table and see where you fit in.

| Effective Preparation | Ineffectual Preparation |
| --- | --- |
| Subscribing to an online question bank and getting through it at least once or twice a week. | Subscribing to an online question bank and getting through 40 percent of it. |
| Buying selective content review books and using them to fill in the knowledge gaps. | Buying selective content review books and stacking them on the floor to collect dust. |
| Writing up missed questions from the online question bank to help you assess and do something about your weak subject areas. | Going through the online question bank and not taking any notes on what was missed. |

| Effective Preparation | Ineffectual Preparation |
|---|---|
| Planning ahead and carving out time to study for Step 1. | Planning on winging the exam. |
| Seeing someone about your suspected test anxiety problem. | Not seeing anyone about your suspected test anxiety problem. |
| Getting tested for a suspected learning disability. | Not getting tested for a suspected learning disability; denying the possibility. |
| Taking the recommendations of your Committee On Student Progress (or equivalent) seriously. | Blowing off the recommendations of your Committee On Student Progress (or equivalent). |

## "Back In The Saddle Again"

Gene Autry's old cowboy song "Back In The Saddle Again" made a comeback in the movie *Sleepless In Seattle*. This song can have many meanings, but the one I like the best is it's time to pick yourself up, dust yourself off, and go for it again. We've all had disappointments and failures in life; it's what you do about them that makes the difference. In the words of Mary Pickford, Oscar-winning Canadian silent-film star and, with other Hollywood movers and shakers Charlie Chaplin, Douglas Fairbanks, and D. W. Griffith, co-founder of United Artists, "If you have made mistakes, even serious mistakes, there is always another chance for you....

for this thing that we call 'failure' is not the falling down, but the staying down." It's time to pick yourself up by the boot-straps. Staying down is not an option if you're serious about passing your Step 1 exam.

## No Guarantees in Life

I wish I could promise that everyone who uses this system will pass, but I can't—there are too many variables. My students have achieved great success, some of which may be due to the structured one-on-one coaching I've provided, but the majority of the credit goes to the students. They did the work, they made the commitment, and they had the courage to try a different approach. Most of them have improved their scores using the AIM YOUR BRAIN Study System. Because of this experience, if one of my students fails Step 1 after work-ing the AIM YOUR BRAIN program, then something else is usually going on. In the past that something else has shown itself to be anxiety that while minimized was actually closer to debilitating test anxiety, an undiagnosed learning disabil-ity, or a combination of both.

If you are feeling that you've done everything you can and are looking for something else, then it may be time to try one of the intensive review courses such as the Cognitive Processing-Based Review for USMLE, Step 1 (CPR-1) at Rosa-lind Franklin University of Medicine and Science, which is in North Chicago (Google search terms = **cpr-1 and Rosalind Franklin**); or the University of Missouri at Kansas City, Insti-tute for Professional Preparation Medical Students (USMLE Step 1 and NBOME COMLEX). Their website is **www.umkc. edu/ipp/usmle-step1.html**. This can be very costly. Travel, food, local transportation, housing, and tuition can cost over

$10,000, but if this is what needs to be done, then it's important for you to look into these programs as well as others that may be available. If you're going to use this book to prepare now (or again) then read on.

## Preparation and Tenacity

The obvious question is what do I do now? The answer is simple. If you picked up this book because you failed Step 1 and are only reading this appendix, then you need to start at the beginning of the book. If you've glanced at this book because someone recommended it, but you're still too shocked by your failure of Step 1, then you, too, need to start at the beginning. If you've used this book before, but really didn't get it or apply it thoroughly, then you need to start at the beginning again and try to figure out what went wrong. Usually, the main problem areas are no time, inadequate preparation, procrastination, unrecognized test anxiety, or an undiagnosed learning disability. I've had students with each of these problems, and I'm happy to say that eventually most passed their USMLE Step 1. Our Committee on Student Progress directed a few students to me. I came into their lives after the remediation plan had been pretty well set. I give you a stylized version of one of these stories in appendix 3.

# APPENDIX 3

# Real-life Successes

## Real-life Student Stories

The stories about Julia and James are based on factual information. One had difficulty preparing for and passing her USMLE Step 1 exam, and the other had concerns about how he should plan and maximize his study effort. I have purposely changed the students' names and background information (family history, gender, etc.) in order to protect their identity. Someday, I hope they can write their own first-person stories to be included in a future revision of this book or as part of an educational website. Many of my students would be willing to write their own stories, but at the moment I'm not comfortable asking them to. I'm probably going overboard, but for now I feel it's the right thing to do. This is the first edition of the book, and some of my former students are still in training.

Both of Julia's parents were doctors, and Julia was destined to follow in their footsteps. Sadly, during college, Julia lost her mother due to illness. Julia knew firsthand about the preciousness of life, and continued her studies with even more determination. While an undergraduate, Julia realized just how much she disliked multiple-choice exams. She excelled at oral and essay examinations but not at timed standardized tests. Despite this, Julia graduated from an excellent California university, passed her MCATs, and was accepted into medical school.

Julia's study methods, which worked quite well during her undergrad years, weren't working as well in medical school. Since a majority of her exams were multiple-choice and, of course, timed, she noticed that it took longer for her to finish tests than it took many of her classmates.

She took her USMLE Step 1 exam and failed it. Devastated by this, she came to me for help. We got to know each other better and worked on preparing her to retake Step 1. After talking to Julia about her difficulties, I was concerned that she might have a learning disability. It wasn't easy, but I was able to talk Julia into getting tested. As it turned out, she did have a learning disability, and the news was hard for her to accept. With time, and using many of the suggestions given to her by the educational psychologist, Julia did great. She worked all of the steps of the AIM YOUR BRAIN Study System (though I hadn't yet given the system that name). Julia passed her Step 1 retake as well as all her other graduation requirements. She graduated and went on to her desired residency program in Southern California.

James heard about my coaching from a friend of his whom I had helped. James had no academic difficulty during his first two years. He was a planner, and just wanted to make sure that he was as prepared as he could be before taking his Step 1. James embraced the AIM YOUR BRAIN Study System wholeheartedly. He dove into his online question bank, wrote up the wrongs, continued to use the F.A.C.T.O.I.D. book he had started, and easily passed Step 1. He went on to pass all of his shelf exams and his remaining USMLE Step 2 CK and CS. He did a great job. He chose to take a year off to do research, and will be a competitive candidate for the National Resident Matching Program.

These are just two stories. There are many more. I'm sure you have your own. Julia and James represent the kinds of issues that many students struggle with, not only at our school, but nationwide and worldwide. If you see any aspect of yourself here, then you need to read on.

## Is There Hope For Me?

I guess I'm an eternal optimist. I see the glass half full rather than half empty. My colleagues in our department will, for the most part, attest to this. I haven't really given up on anyone who was committed to doing the work. To be honest, I did fire a student who didn't do the work. He later wanted to be reinstated and I continued to see him. He had a Step 2 issue. He took the exam before graduation and moved away to start a residency. I don't know whether he was successful. Those were the days when you only had to *take* Step 2 for graduation; now you have to pass it.

I believe there's hope for almost everyone reading this book. I would love to say "everyone" unequivocally, but I don't want to make a promise I might be unable to keep. Everyone is different. I've been fortunate to have motivated students who committed to the program. You, too, can be one of these students by reading this book. I've written it because I know there are a lot of students out there who can benefit from my AIM YOUR BRAIN Study System. There *is* hope for you if you'll do the work and eliminate all of your prior obstacles — inadequate preparation, lack of time, procrastination, etc.

## "Pay It Forward"

My students often ask, "Do they pay you extra to do this?" At the time of this writing, the answer is no. I am a salaried employee of the University of California with other full-time responsibilities. I carve out time to meet with my students during my administration time, before clinics, after clinics, etc. Luckily I have the support of my department chairman and our practice manager.

My students sometimes feel bad because they worry about me staying to meet with them after a long day's work. I tell them it's fine. I do, however, ask one thing of them in return: I ask them to pay it forward.

The phrase "pay it forward" is based on the fiction book written by Catherine Ryan Hyde. It was also released as a movie in 2000. Trevor, the hero of the book and movie, comes up with an idea. In essence, he does something good for three other people, and instead of getting paid back for his good work, he tells them to "pay it forward." In other words, the people he helped have to help three more people, and so on. Catherine Ryan Hyde has actually started a foundation based on this theme.

My concept of paying it forward is simple. I just ask my students as they become interns, residents, attendings, faculty, etc., to help the students they come across just as they were helped. Since I've tried to keep the names of the students I work with confidential, I don't routinely ask them to help their peers, but once in a great while, I may have a student who could benefit from a firsthand description of the experience of a student who has already gone through a similar challenge. My students have been great! When I've called a senior student to ask if he or she would be willing to speak to another student, the answer has been yes. I get permission from both students to arrange the phone call and disclose names. I give them each other's phone numbers and tell them who will be calling whom. Then I stay out of it.

Deciding to write this book is my way to pay it forward on a larger scale. I'm just one person, and experience has shown me that the need for help in studying for Step 1 is growing. The best thing I can do is write the book and get the website going. Please just remember to pay it forward as you move along in your career.

## Your Future in Medicine, Exams, and the AIM YOUR BRAIN Study System

If you find success using the AIM YOUR BRAIN Study System, I believe it will help you as you encounter more and more multiple-choice tests in your training, in-service exams, and specialty boards (yes, I've helped a few students pass their specialty boards as well).

The most important thing you can do is remember to use it. If you've always had problems with multiple-choice questions, I'm sorry to tell you that situation isn't going away. What's different is that you now have a system, an approach, that you can use to deal with them. You'll need to get lots of study questions and work through them (don't forget to time yourself). You'll need to write up the wrongs in a F.A.C.T.O.I.D. book so you can see firsthand your areas of weakness and do something about them. You'll need to review your F.A.C.T.O.I.D. book(s) over and over again. You'll need to go through your timed question sets again. You'll need to pay attention to interruptions, setting aside enough time to study, and deal with any feelings of test anxiety. If you have a learning disability or debilitating test anxiety (DTA), you may need to do more.

I believe that if the AIM YOUR BRAIN Study System has been successful for you in the past, it can work for you again in the future. If you need to tweak it a little, then tweak it a little. Thanks for reading the book. Don't forget to visit our website www.ideas2pen.com for the latest and greatest information. Remember: you *can* do it!

# Notes

1.  Hubbard, J. P. and E. J. Levit. *The National Board of Medical Examiners: the first seventy years; a continuing commitment to excellence.* Philadelphia: The Board, 1985.

2.  *Educational Commission for Foreign Medical Graduates 2002 Annual Report.* April 18, 2003 [cited 2007 January 28]; Available from www.ecfmg.org/annuals/2002/history.html.

3.  Hallock, J. A. Viewpoint: "In Golden Anniversary and Beyond, Collaboration is Key." *AAMC Reporter*: September 2006 [cited 2006 December 16]; Available from www.aamc.org/newsroom/reporter/sept06/viewpoint.htm.

4.  Merritt, S. Mastering Multiple Choice, in *The Definitive Guide to Better Grades on Multiple Choice Exams.* Brain Ranch, 2006.

5.  Multiple-choice, in Dictionary.com, Unabridged. Random House, Inc. 2006.

6.  Hubbard, J. P., Measuring medical education; the tests and test procedures of the National Board of Medical Examiners. Philadelphia: Lea & Febiger, 1971.

7.  Hubbard, J. P. and W. V. Clemans. Multiple-choice examinations in medicine, a guide for examiner and examinee. Philadelphia: Lea & Febiger, 1961.

8.  FSMB and NBME. USMLE examinations. 1996–2009 **http://www.usmle.org/examinations/step1/step1-test.html**.

9.  Goldsmith, C. and J. Katz. Transmission electron micrograph (TEM), taken at a magnification of 108,000×, revealed the ultrastructural details of two avian influenza A (H5N1) virions. CDC.

10. Brown, S. This photomicrograph of a vaginal smear identifies *Candida albicans* while using a wet mount technique. CDC, 1976.

11. NBME. Annual Report. Message from the President 2004 [cited 2006 December 26, 2006]; Available from www.nbme.org/AnnualReport/2004/highlights.htm.

12. Learn, in Dictionary.com Unabridged. Random House, Inc., 2006

13. Feat, in *The American Heritage Dictionary of the English Language.* Houghton Mifflin Company, 2004.

14. Meier, D. *The Accelerated Learning Handbook.* New York: The McGraw-Hill Companies, 2000. 274.

15. Walsh, B. E., *Unleashing Your Brilliance.* 2005, Victoria, BC: Walsh Seminars Ltd. 274.

16. Sight, in Dictionary.com Unabridged. Random House, Inc., 2006

17. Sound, in Dictionary.com Unabridged. Random House, Inc., 2006

18. Motion, in Dictionary.com Unabridged. Random House, Inc., 2006

19. Muse, in Dictionary.com Unabridged. Random House, Inc., 2006

20. Ariniello, L., Blood Brain Barrier. Society for Neuroscience: Brain Briefings, 1999.

21. FDA, Drugs used in the treatment of HIV infection. 2008.

22. CDC, Influenza viruses. 2005(The Virus & Its Spread).

23. WHO, Avian influenza ("bird flu") - Fact sheet, 2006.

24. CDC, Diseases Characterized by Vaginal Discharge. Sexually Transmitted Diseases Treatment Guidelines 2006, 2006.

25. Tracy, B. *Eat That Frog! 21 great ways to stop procrastinating and get more done in less time.* San Francisco: Berrett-Koehler Publishers, Inc., 2007.

26. procrastination. *The American Heritage Dictionary of the English Language, 4th ed.* Houghton Mifflin Company, 2004.

27. Self-discipline. *The American Heritage Dictionary of the English Language, 4th ed.* Houghton Mifflin Company, 2004.

28. Oldenburg, R. *The Great Good Place: Cafes, coffee shops, bookstores, bars, hair salons and other hangouts at the heart of a community.* New York: Marlowe and Company, 1999.

29. King, S. On Writing: A memoir of the craft. New York: Scribner, 2000.

30. Spielberger, C. D. and P. R. Vagg. Test Anxiety Theory, assessment, and treatment. The Series In Clinical and Community Psychology. Washington, DC: Taylor & Francis, 1995.

31. Powell, D. H. Behavioral treatment of debilitating test anxiety among medical students. J Clin Psychol, 2004. 60(8): p. 853–65.

32. Bandura, A. *Self-Efficacy: The Exercise of Control.* New York: W. H. Freeman and Company, 1997.

33. Birk, L. Pharmacotherapy for performance anxiety disorders: occasionally useful but typically contraindicated. *J Clin Psychol,* 2004. 60(8): p. 867–79.

34. Powell, D. H. Treating individuals with debilitating performance anxiety: An introduction. *J Clin Psychol,* 2004. 60(8): p. 801–8.

35. Talisman, in Dictionary.com Unabridged. Random House, Inc., 2006.

36. Courage, in Dictionary.com Unabridged. Random House, Inc., 2006.

37. Perseverance, in Dictionary.com Unabridged. Random House, Inc., 2006.

38. Boylan, Bob. *What's Your Point? The 3-Step Method for Making Effective Presentations.* New York: Warner Books, Inc., 1988.

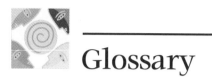

# Glossary

**AAMC:** Association of American Medical Colleges

**AHA:** American Hospital Association

**AIM YOUR BRAIN** Study System: The method describe in this book that transforms concepts into little bits of information that can get in and out of your brain quickly and efficiently during multiple-choice exams.

**allopathic medical students:** Students enrolled in an M.D. medical school.

**AMA:** American Medical Association.

**AOA:** American Osteopathic Association.

**blocked-brain barrier:** A condition in which a student knows the material or subject matter, but just can't get it out quickly and accurately enough on timed multiple-choice exams.

**blood-brain barrier:** A specialized barrier in the brain that protected its cells.

**CBT:** Computer-based testing.

**CCGFMS:** Cooperating Committee on Graduates of Foreign Medical Schools.

**courage:** Mental or moral strength to venture, persevere, and withstand danger, fear, or difficulty.

**crisis management:** The act or practice of dealing with a crisis when it develops.

**distracters:** Alternative responses or completions in a multiple-choice question, which are incorrect.

**DO:** Doctor of Osteopathic Medicine.

**DTA:** Debilitating test anxiety.

**ECFMG:** Educational Commission for Foreign Medical Graduates.

**exam postmortem:** The process of trying to figure out what you did right and what you did wrong after taking an examination.

**Exam Master:** Online question bank company.

**F.A.C.T.O.I.D.®:** Frequently Asked Concepts To Own In-Depth.

**F.A.C.T.O.I.D.® book:** A single-subject spiral-bound note-book that holds notes (written in a special format) on missed questions and used for review.

**faculty coach:** Your faculty coach should be someone you can trust; who you will be accountable to; and someone who will guide you.

**feat:** An act of skill, endurance, imagination, or strength; an achievement.

**feats of learning:** Acquiring knowledge by studying skillfully.

**Form 990:** The annual return for tax-exempt organizations.

**FSMB:** Federation of State Medical Boards.

**green sheet:** Plain 3 × 4-inch tablets that have my name, department, and phone number. I started using them because they were handy and plentiful.

**IMG:** International medical graduate.

**interruption:** Some abrupt occurrence that interrupts an ongoing activity.

**Kaplan:** Online question-bank company.

**LCME:** Liaison Committee on Medical Education.

**learn:** To acquire knowledge of or skill in by study, instruction, or experience.

**learning preference:** How you learn best: sight, sound, motion, or muse.

**MCQ:** Multiple-choice question.

**M.D.:** Doctor of Medicine.

**mock schedule:** Sample schedule.

**motion:** The action or process of moving or of changing place or position; movement.

**MP3:** A file extension for compressed MPEG-3 audio files.

**MP4:** A file extension for compressed MPEG-4 audio and video files.

**muse:** To think or meditate in silence, as on some subject.

**multiple-choice question:** A question consisting of several possible answers from which the correct one must be selected.

**multiple-choice test:** An exam made up of multiple-choice questions.

**NBME:** National Board of Medical Examiners.

**online question banks:** Questions banks maintained by companies that allow online access.

**pay it forward:** The concept of helping future students with their test-taking challenges when a former student becomes an intern, resident, or attending physician.

**perseverance:** Steady persistence in a course of action, a purpose, a state, etc., esp. in spite of difficulties, obstacles, or discouragement.

**Pinocchio nose:** A reference to the Pinocchio children's story and how the puppet character's nose would grow when he didn't tell the truth.

**PPT:** Pen-and-paper test.

**Princeton Review:** Online question bank company.

**procrastination:** To put off doing something, especially out of habitual carelessness or laziness.

**Prometric:** Test centers used for USMLE.

**pseudo-faculty coach:** Friends or family who end up filling the role of a faculty coach.

**psychologist:** A person trained and educated to perform psychological research, testing, and therapy.

**quatrain:** A four-line poem that often rhymes.

**review books:** Books usually purchased, borrowed from friends, or checked out from the library to help with course or exam content preparation.

**rock bottom:** A metaphor for trying to assess unrecognized areas of content weakness.

**SAFETI:** Safety Abroad First Educational Travel Information.

**SAVI:** An acronym for the learning preferences, somatic, auditory, visual, and intellectual, developed by Dave Meier.

**self-discipline:** Training and control of oneself and one's conduct, usually for personal improvement.

**self-talk:** The internal dialogue people use to communicate within themselves.

**sight:** The power or faculty of seeing; perception of objects by use of the eyes; vision.

**S.O.:** Significant other.

**sound:** The sensation produced by stimulation of the organs of hearing by vibrations transmitted through the air or other medium.

**standardized test:** Usually a commercially developed test administered and scored in a uniform or consistent manner.

**stem:** The portion of a multiple-choice question which actually asks the question, makes a statement, poses a problem involving images, charts or graphs, or presents a case history.

**Step 1:** The first step of a three-part written exam series that focuses on the things learned during the first two years of medical school, i.e., basic sciences.

**Sudoku:** A logic-based number-placement puzzle.

**tag:** A tag is a (relevant) keyword or term associated with or assigned to a piece of information (e.g., a picture, article, or video clip), thus describing the item and enabling keyword-based classification of information.

**talisman:** Anything whose presence exercises a remarkable or powerful influence on human feeling or actions.

**test anxiety:** A situation-specific anxiety trait that involves the frequency and intensity of the emotional reactions and worry cognitions students experience during examinations.

**test rehearsal:** The pre-exam version of a dress rehearsal designed to work out bugs and make any last minute changes, learn about the test center, and reduce as much anxiety as possible.

**third place:** A place of solitude, not comradery.

**three-digit scale:** The usual USMLE score format students use to convey their test results.

**two-digit scale:** Other reporting format for USMLE score.

**USD:** United States dollars.

**USMLE:** United States Medical Licensing Examination.

**Usmleworld.com:** Online question bank company.

**visualization:** A special place students can go to "in their minds" to help center themselves.

**white space:** One line of space between similar concepts, two lines of space between new concepts, at least to help make F.A.C.T.O.I.D. book reviews more tolerable and less dense.

**workload:** The amount of work assigned to or expected of a worker in a specified time period.

# Index

# About the Author

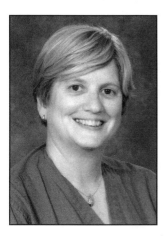

**Dr. Miller** is a Clinical Professor and Clinic Medical Director for the Ellison Ambulatory and Cypress Clinics in the Department of Obstetrics and Gynecology at the University of California, Davis–School of Medicine. She is also the ombudsperson for the 3rd- and 4th-year medical students. Dr. Miller is a graduate of Michigan State University, College of Human Medicine (M.D.), and a graduate of the University of the Pacific, School of Pharmacy (Pharm.D.) She has won numerous national teaching awards including APGO (Association of Professors of Gynecology and Obstetrics), CREOG (Council on Resident Education in Obstetrics and Gynecology), and the Kaiser Foundation Award for Excellence in Teaching. She is also the author of *Mathematics For Nurses With Clinical Applications* (Brooks/Cole Publishing). Dr. Miller lives in northern California and loves to dance, listen to music, ride recumbent trikes (and crank-forward bikes), fiddle with techie gadgets, and snorkel.

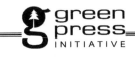
**green press** INITIATIVE

Ideas2Pen is committed to preserving ancient forests and natural resources. We elected to print *AIM YOUR BRAIN at USMLE Step 1* on 30% post consumer recycled paper, processed chlorine-free.

As a result, for this printing, we have saved:

  12 trees (40' tall, 6-8" in diameter)

  2,662 gallons of water

  5 million BTUs of total energy

  342 pounds of solid waste

  641 pounds of greenhouse gases

Ideas2Pen made this choice because we are a member of Green Press Initiative, a nonprofit program dedicated to supporting authors, publishers, and suppliers in their efforts to reduce their use of fiber obtained from endangered forests.

For more information, visit
www.greenpressinitiative.org

Calculations from www.papercalculator.org